MCQ TUTOR.
PSYCHIATRY

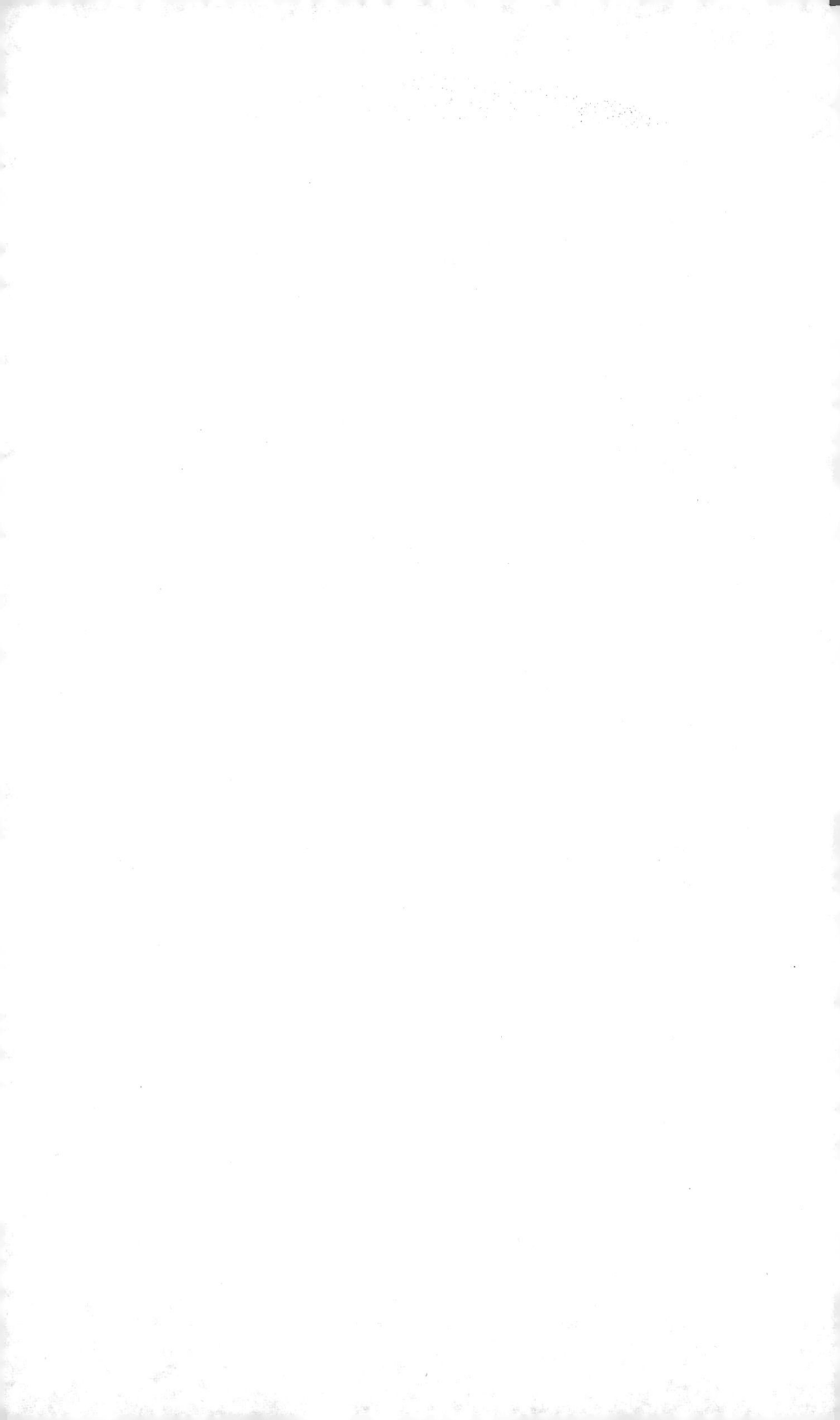

MCQ TUTOR: PSYCHIATRY

Michael A. Simpson, M.B., B.S., M.R.C.S., M.R.C. Psych., D.P.M.
Professor of Psychiatry, University of the Orange Free State, South Africa

Formerly:
Professor of Psychiatry
Professor of Family Practice & Community Health,
Temple University, Philadelphia, Pennsylvania, U.S.A.

WILLIAM HEINEMANN MEDICAL BOOKS LTD
London

First published 1983

© Michael A. Simpson

ISBN 0-433-30340-9

Filmset by Reproduction Drawings Ltd., Sutton, Surrey
Printed in Great Britain by Spottiswoode Ballantyne Ltd.,
Colchester and London

Dedicated to Peggy,
for your everlasting, invaluable support and help.

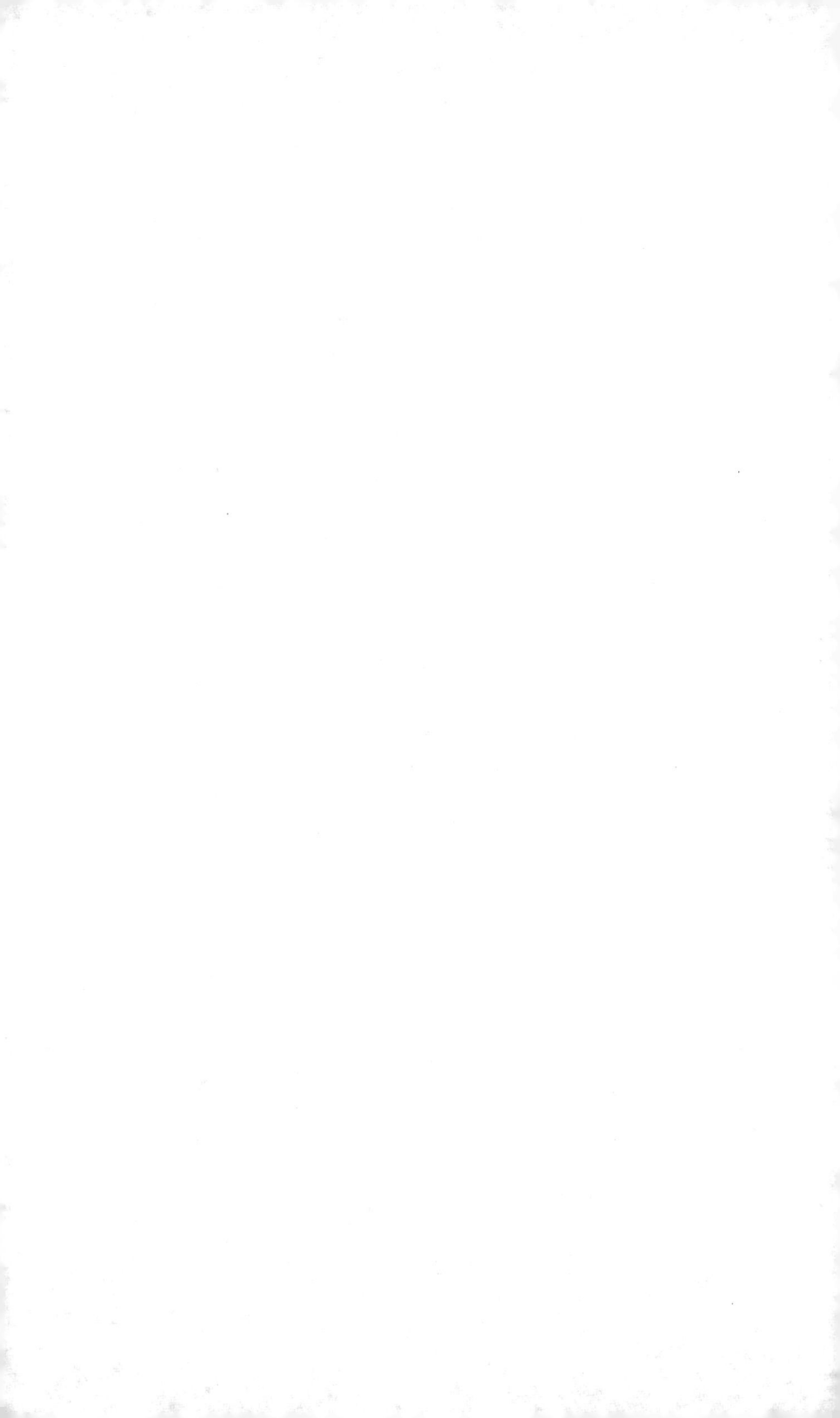

INTRODUCTION

'Examinations are formidable even to the best prepared, for the greatest fool may ask more than the wisest man can answer,' said Charles Kaleb Colton. Few statements are both so true and so comforting to the examination candidate, and so usefully cautionary for the examiner.

This self-tutor book is intended to help you learn psychiatry, and to assess the extent to which your studies have been successful. It will be useful for medical students, though it is tailored especially for the needs of candidates preparing for higher specialty examinations in psychiatry—particularly the British M.R.C. Psych. (the Preliminary Test and the Membership Examination), the American Specialty Boards, and the equivalent examinations in Australia, New Zealand and Canada. The questions cover the range of subjects required for these examinations. In the M.R.C. Psych. preliminary test, for example, this includes:

i) Structure, functions and pathology of the nervous system with reference to psychiatry (including basic and applied neuroanatomy, neurophysiology, biochemistry and neuroendocrinology, and the action of drugs on the central nervous system);
ii) genetics applied to psychiatry;
iii) psychology applied to psychiatry (including experimental, clinical, developmental and social psychology and ethology);
iv) basic clinical psychopathology (descriptive, experimental, dynamic and phenomenological); and
v) methodology of investigations in psychiatry (including elementary statistics and epidemiology).

In the M.R.C. Psych. Membership examination, the subjects include:

i) aspects of general medicine as applied to psychiatry;
ii) manifestations of psychiatric disorders in children, adults and the aged in their clinical and community aspects;
iii) aspects of epidemiology relevant to psychiatry;
iv) history of psychiatry.

The questions in this book will not be presented in separate sections arranged by topic, but mixed, as they are in actual postgraduate examinations. There is a separate subject index which will enable you to identify questions by subject, if you wish to test yourself in specific subject areas.

The answers are given on the page following the questions. Where appropriate, there is a discussion of the answers, to explain them more fully. In some instances, where further discussion would not be profitable, or where the issues are discussed elsewhere, such discussion will be minimal or absent.

When it would be useful there are references to specific articles, good reviews or sections of current textbooks. Two most recent competent textbooks have been used for multiple references: *CTP* refers to the *Modern Synopsis of the Comprehensive Textbook of Psychiatry III* by H I Kaplan and B J Sadock, 3rd edition, Williams & Wilkins, Baltimore & London, 1981; and *CPM* refers to *Clinical Psychiatric Medicine* by A E Slaby, L R Tancredi and J Lieb. Harper & Row, Philadelphia, 1981. *GP* refers to *Guide to Psychiatry* by Myre Sim, 4th edition, Churchhill–Livingstone, London, 1981, and is the current British text used.

MULTIPLE-CHOICE QUESTIONS

However ambivalent we may feel about Multiple Choice Questions (MCQ's), they are likely to remain in use and are generally more fair to the candidate than most believe. They provide a reasonably reliable measure of knowledge across a wide field, reducing the effects of examiner idiosyncracy. They are intended to produce results influenced only by the factors they are designed to test. Unlike other techniques, they can be applied equally to large numbers of candidates at one time, and they are relatively easy for MCQ papers to be marked automatically and scored by computer. This allows the results to be analyzed, not only to assess the candidate, but also to assess the examination itself, to identify and reject ambiguous or unfair questions.

As there are several types of MCQ, get to know the particular format used in the examination you are to sit. The Royal College of Psychiatrists (which provides a sample preliminary test paper) uses the most basic type. Each question consists of an initial statement (or stem) followed by a number of completions (or items), usually five, identified by the letters (a) (b) (c) (d) and (e). Usually a question has both true and false items, though it may contain all true or false items.

Get to know the marking system being used, as this will affect your strategies. You will need to know if there is a penalty for guessing (deductions of marks for wrong answers), and, if so, how severe is the penalty. In some systems there is no penalty or counter-mark, and of course one should answer every question and guess even where one has absolutely no idea of the right answer. In others, one scores +1 for each correct answer, and −1 for wrong answers. Another common system, used by the Royal College of Psychiatrists, is to give 1/n marks (where n is the number of items within the question) for each item correctly identified as true or false; and to deduct 1/n marks for each item incorrectly identified; while items left blank do not influence the score at all. Thus, on a question with five alternative answers, you would score 0.2 marks for each item correctly identified, and lose 0.2 marks for each wrong identification. Correctly identifying all five items on the question would result in a score of 1 mark.

The idea of counter-marking is to discourage guessing, which is unfortunate for, in much of medicine, informed and educated guessing is exactly what is needed, and few decisions are ever made with certainty. It was assumed that penalizing wrong answers would discourage guessing and let the test reflect more clearly what the candidate actually knows. In fact, fear of losing points inhibits most people from answering items they do know, but about which they do not feel fully confident. In fact, it is more likely to produce divergence between candidates on the basis of how prepared they are to take risks, rather than by knowledge. Fortunately, in most cases, it is still profitable to guess intelligently. While one cannot pass an exam without knowledge of the subject, intelligent strategy can maximize the score one does achieve. Harden and others have pointed out that with the +1, −1, 0 marking scheme, candidates improved their marks when they went back over a paper and answered the uncertain questions they had previously left blank.

In systems with no counter-marking, like the American Boards, where your score is the sum of the total number of test items you answer right, you *must* guess and answer every item. Even a random guess has a 20% chance of being right in a five option MCQ. If you do not have time to finish the test, at least put random answers to every question. With most counter-marking systems it is still profitable to answer all questions, even if one must guess some answers. As you rarely know absolutely nothing about a topic, and may be able to eliminate at least one or two of the possibilities, your probability of guessing correctly is usually better than pure chance. The British Royal College of Psychiatrists' system discourages random guessing, but it is still worth answering all items where you have some knowledge.

In the Exam

You will have prepared properly. It is not a good idea to spend the night before the exam doing anything distracting. It is best to either have an early night and get some good rest, or, if it makes you feel more secure, to study late or even through the night. There are no pharmacological aids to learning, but remember the phenomena of state-dependent learning. If you use something like caffeine to help you stay awake to study, do not attempt to take the exam while deprived of caffeine. Do not spend the last few minutes before the exam swapping questions with other candidates—you will probably only frighten each other. Do not try and pack in extra new information. If you want to study up to the last minute, take some very familiar summary notes of your own.

Arrive well-equipped, with a pen, a couple of good sharp 2B pencils, an eraser, and a reliable watch.

Read the instructions carefully and make quite sure you understand what you are being asked to do. Check, even if you've taken the test before—there may have been changes since last time.

Scan through the questions quickly, just to get a brief overall picture of what to expect, and develop a rough time-table for the exam and budget your time. You will probably have up to one minute per question. Never spend too much time on any one question or item, because it will reduce the time you have available for other questions. If you 'block' or cannot remember an item, or have trouble with one group of questions, mark the spot in the question paper, move on and come back to them later. Above all, do not panic. A temporary lapse of memory is perfectly normal and common, but will only get worse if you worry about it too much. Have realistic expectations of yourself. No one scores 100% on a major, standardized MCQ examination: they are not designed for most people to be able to answer everything correctly. If everyone scored 100%, we would have to start all over again!

So if you have to miss out some items or questions, you will have plenty of company, and can still pass the examination. But if you let yourself get too upset by what you don't know, you may get anxious enough to forget what you do know.

Mark your answers clearly on the answer sheet, with a firm clear pencil mark in the appropriate box. All these points may seem very obvious, but they are commonly neglected. People fail exams by marking the right answers in the wrong boxes. One can easily skip a question and then begin to write the answer to question 46 as a response to question 45 or 47, throwing all subsequent answers out. It is not a good idea to note your answers on the question paper and then transfer them to the answer sheet. This takes extra time you may not be able to afford, and increases your chances of marking the answers down incorrectly.

The commonest type of question you will meet will be the standard or A-type question, as described above. Some authors suggest that one may find clues to the right answers in the questions. Such clues may include a relationship apparent between the stem and the correct option by repetition of words or parts of a word; the use of an absurd option where the question writer is having difficulty constructing plausible alternatives; the correct answer being longer (occasionally shorter) than the alternatives (distractors) or identifiable by over-generalization or over-qualification. There is a tendency among test-writers to put the right answer in the same place (for example, quite often as alternative (c)) over a series of questions. In professional examinations this will have been corrected, as has been done in this book, where the correct answers have been carefully allocated at random between different positions.

Do not worry about items that seem to be bad questions, just answer them as best you can. Item analysis during the scoring will show which are poor items, and they will be eliminated from scores. Do not choose a time like this to quarrel with the examiners, or get angry—this is one time when one does not win such arguments. With a good scoring system, one would not need to.

Do not leave early. If you finish with time to spare, check your answers again. Do not change your answers too readily, however, unless you have good reason to do so. Your first guess is probably more reliable than subsequent guesses—except when subsequent questions have given you good clues for revisions.

By and large, you can trust the examiner. Accept the questions as they stand, without too much quibbling. They have tried to remove ambiguities—do not search for hidden meanings or clever catches. Only a very stupid examiner tries to ask trick questions. Do not invent difficulties. The obvious meaning of the statements is what is meant. 'Commonly', 'characteristic', 'recognized effects', 'are associated with' and 'typical of' are words or phrases often used in questions. A *characteristic* feature is one that occurs often, and is of diagnostic significance, such that its absence might cast some doubt on the diagnosis. It may not be an exclusive feature, but is *typical*. A *recognized* effect may not be strictly 'characteristic' but is one that has been generally reported to occur, and would be known and agreed by most clinicians in the field. (What is 'characteristic' would, necessarily, be 'recognized'; what is 'recognized' as occurring in a condition, might not be 'characteristic'). *Pathognomic* or *specific* features are those which occur in the condition named, and in no other.

Other, vaguer terms are sometimes used, like 'often' or 'commonly' (as well as 'sometimes', 'frequently', 'routine', 'rare', etc.) but one tends to avoid them. How common is common? Where these terms are used, take a common-sense interpretation.

A common alternative format, popular in American examinations, is the K-type MCQ. A typical question would be:

Depression may be caused by

1) Methyldopa
2) Frusemide
3) Reserpine
4) Dothiepin

The instructions would point out that one or more of the options is correct and to mark (a) if you believe that only 1,2, and 3 are correct; (b) if only 1 and 3 are right; (c) if 2 and 4 are right; (d) if only 4 is correct; and (e) if all are correct.

Despite their apparent complexity, these are not hard to deal with. Concentrate on the four numbered options and see how many you can eliminate as false. If you can rule out even one of them, there are only two possible answers to the question left so even a blind guess has a 50% chance of being right. If, in this example, you are sure dothiepin, as an antidepressant, does not cause depression, you have ruled out answers (c), (d) and (e), all of which need (4) to be correct. The right answer has to be (a) or (b). In fact, you can now be sure that options (1) and (3) are right, as they are contained in both the remaining options, and your choice will depend on whether (2) is true or false.

Watch out for negatively phrased questions, like 'All of the following are tricyclics EXCEPT', or 'which of the following is/are *not* tricyclic?', and avoid answering them as if they were positively phrased.

Give the answer by the book. Even where you have special experience or knowledge in an area, if you know you opinion varies from the typical or book version, do not give your own idiosyncratic answer. You can write your own book later. Give the examiner what he seems to be looking for.

Some years ago, the author devised the simple technique of the 'Reverse MCQ'. Recognizing the great difficulty of the exercise of writing good MCQ, he would as part of a course evaluation ask the students or residents to write or set four or five multiple choice questions, rather than to answer thirty. It demonstrates an even better understanding of your subject to be able to set good questions than to answer them. It would be a useful exercise for readers to write some MCQ for themselves. They will develop their understanding of the subject, and gain some empathy for the difficulty of the task of the examiner and of this author. Such insight may also be helpful in taking further MCQ examinations.

ORAL AND CLINICAL EXAMINATION

To prepare properly, you need to do more than good basic reading of the standard texts and articles in the subject. It is important to practise for the clinical and oral examinations. Take 30 to 45 minutes to see a new patient, take a history, perform a mental status examination. Then have a colleague or tutor give you a half-hour 'grilling', questioning you about the case and related subjects.

On the day of the exam, it is worth paying attention to your appearance, as it will influence the examiners even though they try to remain objective. They might fairly conclude that a scruffy and disorganized appearance may reflect a scruffy and disorganized manner of practice. Similarly, over-dressing can be distracting. Overtly seductive dress may reflect an attempt to sway the examiners in your favour which if it fails, as it often does (it is not easy to successfully appeal to two examiners at the same time, and unsuccessful seduction is unpopular), it will not help you, and may raise doubts about your mode of clinical practice.

Your accent and manner of expressing yourself will be relevant. Examiners will not and should not be biased for or against particular regional or national accents, and may even over-correct for them. But you must be able to speak comprehensibly. The examiners should expect this, for if they are unable to undersand you when you are trying your best, your patients are unlikely to manage better under ordinary circumstances.

Many foreign medical graduates have problems in this respect, and often fail to realistically attempt to improve their language and expressive skills. Feeling awkward about their fluency, they may avoid opportunities to take part actively in tutorials and discussion groups where they would have a chance to hear and practise speaking colloquial English in relation to their subject. Often, they rely too much on only reading about psychiatry, so they may be familiar with concepts and facts which they have never heard spoken and are unable to discuss.

In the orals and clinicals, the examiner is basically trying to pass people. One is expecting a reasonable standard of competence and expertise, and is well aware of one's duty to protect the public against substandard specialists. But most people after average training, clinical experience and study, should be able to pass. We are not usually trying to fail you. However, we do need data and good reasons to substantiate the decision to pass you. If you take too much time in answering questions, we can ask you less in the time available, and you will have less chance to show how much you know. The bigger the sample of your knowledge we are able to assess, the less important individual wrong answers or uncertainties may be. One mistake out of three questions suggests less familiarity with the topic than three errors out of seventeen questions. In the oral exam, you may be asked if you specialize, and may be questioned about your special field, but the examiners will not confine themselves to that field.

Do not flannel; do not fudge and ramble in an attempt to disguise the fact that you do not know the answer to a question: it is usually obvious that you do not know and it is far more worrying to the examiner if it looks as if you do not know what you do not know! It's far better to admit that you do not know or have forgotten that point and let us proceed to other matters more fruitful for you to discuss. The person who knows what he does not know can learn it; the person who does not know what he does not know is dangerous.

Instructions to the examiners in the American National Boards (2) tell them to 'avoid discussion of abstract, obscure matters of questionable importance. If areas are uncovered in which the candidate is not informed, do not dwell exclusively on these topics. Find out what else he may know.'

Examiners are especially concerned with how a candidate thinks about a patient's problems—how he assesses the situation, and how he makes decisions. It can be very useful for you to give them access to this process. Even where you cannot recall all the relevant facts, you may show how effectively you can use the available information. You can talk openly about how you reached the conclusions you report, and mention other information you may need. If nervousness or lack of time leads you to omit part of the history or examination, it is usually better to mention it as something omitted, but which you would want to know, rather than let the examiner conclude that you would never think of it under normal conditions.

Another instruction to American Boards' examiners states, 'There is no place for sarcasm or humour at the candidate's expense, or attitudes of condescension or cool hostility. Make every effort to put the candidate at ease and to encourage his best performance'. Though some examiners are idiosyncratic in their manner with candidates, much effort is expended to avoid problems, and there are probably more difficulties arising from bizarre behaviour of candidates than from that of examiners. If you are not sure what the examiner wants or what his question means, feel free to ask for clarification.

In the clinical, use your time with the patient well to establish rapport and gather organized clinical data. Introduce yourself and your situation, for example, 'My name is Dr Simpson, and I will be talking with you for about an hour as part of an examination I am taking. How do you feel about my talking with you?' Start with basic demographic data (name, age, work and marital status). Do not feel it inappropriate to ask the patient which doctors he has been seeing and what they said, what diagnosis or what explanation of his symptoms he has been offered, and what treatment he has been receiving.

There has been some concern among candidates about what type of formulation they should offer the examiners. In the M.R.C. Psych. exam, candidates are told: 'A formulation is the candidate's assessment of the case and not just a summary of the facts. It should include a critical discussion of diagnosis, differential diagnosis and possible aetiological factors, together with a plan of management (including investigations) and an estimate of prognosis'. You are not expected to carry out a physical examination routinely, but may do so if you clinical interview leads you to consider it useful. You will have one hour to examine the patient, and 5 minutes to outline your formulation. Then there will be a 30 minute interview with two examiners, devoted to matters relevant to the patient's case. If the examiners wish it, they may ask you to interview the patient again in their presence.

What is a 'formulation'? 'Formulate' is defined in the *Oxford English Dictionary* as 'to reduce to, or express in, a formula; to set forth in a definite and systematic statement.' The Teaching Committee of the Department of Psychiatry at the Institute of Psychiatry, London describes an 'initial formulation' as 'a doctor's assessment of the case rather than a re-statement of the facts.... It should always include a discussion of the diagnosis, the aetiological factors which seem important, as well as taking into account the patient's life situation and background, with a plan of treatment and an estimate of prognosis. Regardless of the uncertainty or complexity of the case, a provisional diagnosis should always be specified.'

A workshop of the Association of Psychiatrists in Training (APIT) suggested that the formulation should review your deductions, based on the information you obtained from the history and examination, and should include:

1) A brief *introduction* to the problem, e.g. 'This is a 27-year-old unemployed male engineer whose main complaint is increasing depression over the past two months'.

2) A *differential diagnosis* reviewing the likely diagnosis and other possibilities in order of importance.
3) A *justification* for your differential diagnosis, including the most significant positive and negative points from the history and examination.
4) A comment on further *investigations* or information you would like to clarify issues such as history from other informants, old charts and notes, physical and psychological investigations.
5) Your *management plans*—would you admit him to hospital? What psychological, pharmacological and other treatment would you propose? What plans have you regarding the family, work, rehabilitation, and long term management.

A recent Royal College of Psychiatrists discussion document summarized the above definitions and suggested that the formulation should summarize 'the relevant genetic, constitutional and personality factors, taking into account the patient's life situation.'

When using this book, make a note of your answers to each question, before turning the page for the answers and discussion. Otherwise it is very easy to convince oneself that one really meant to give the right answers after all, and one may receive an artificially rosy view of one's knowledge. If you want to test yourself in conditions more like an examination, set yourself the task of answering 30, 60 or 90 questions at a time, allowing one minute per question and ignoring the answers until you have completed the set.

I hope you enjoy working through the questions and answers, and exploring some of the references. Suggestions of further questions to use in other editions, would be received with interest.

Philadelphia & London   Michael A. Simpson
1982

1. Which of the following are catecholamines?

   a) Serotonin
   b) Dopa
   c) Dopamine
   d) Noradrenaline
   e) Homovanillic acid

2. Which of the following psychological tests are NOT measures of personality traits or factors?

   a) The E.P.I.
   b) The M.M.P.I.
   c) The 16–PF
   d) The Bannister–Fransella Repertory Grid
   e) Progressive Matrices

3. Thickening of peripheral nerves may be apparent on palpation in each of the following conditions, EXCEPT:

   a) Vitamin deficiency
   b) Leprosy
   c) Carpal tunnel syndrome in acromegaly
   d) Amyloidosis
   e) Hypertrophic interstitial neuritis

Answers overleaf

1. c), d)

Dopamine and noradrenaline are catecholamines. Homovanillic acid is one of the neurotransmitter metabolites of dopamine. Serotonin and dopa are not catecholamines.

CTP Chap. 2.2, pp. 41–5. *CPM* Chap. 3, Chap. 7, pp. 133–6. *GP* pp. 515–16.

2. d), e)

The Eysenck Personality Inventory (EPI) describes personality in terms of neuroticism, extraversion and psychoticism. The Minnesota Multiphasic Personality Inventory (MMPI) produces scores on various scales describing psychiatrically oriented personality aspects such as depression, paranoia, hysteria, etc. The 16-Personality Factor (16-PF) instrument estimates personality traits like self-sufficiency, submissiveness, and imaginativeness. The grid (e) measures how integrated and consistent one's thinking is, and may be useful in identifying schizophrenic thought disorder. The Progressive Matrices are an intelligence test, sensitive to demonstrating intellectual deterioration.

CTP, Chap. 10.5, pp. 214–6, 10.7 pp. 216–1. *GP* pp. 9–16.

3. a)

Such thickening is not typical of vitamin deficiency, though it is seen in all the other conditions mentioned.

Brain W.R. (1955)

4. The only tricyclic antidepressant for which a 'therapeutic window' effect has been convincingly shown to exist, relating plasma levels to therapeutic efficacy, is:

   a) Amitriptyline
   b) Nortriptyline
   c) Imipramine
   d) Desipramine
   e) Doxepin

5. In managing the suicidal patient, the therapist should:

   a) Delay the relief of symptoms to encourage motivation for treatment
   b) Be more active than usual in developing a therapeutic relationship with the patient
   c) Be more passive and reflective in relating to the patient
   d) Minimize or if possible avoid contact with the patient's family
   e) None of the above

6. Which of the following psychotropic drugs is safe to prescribe during lactation?

   a) Meprobamate
   b) Diazepam
   c) Chlordiazepoxide
   d) Amitriptyline
   e) None of the above

Answers overleaf

4. b)

Though further exploration is needed, only for nortriptyline has the so-called 'therapeutic window' effect been convincingly demonstrated. Not only is the drug not clinically effective *below* a certain plasma level, but it also loses efficacy *above* a certain plasma level (the levels are around 50–150 ng/ml).

Silverman J. J., *et al.* (1979).
CTP Chap. 29.2 p. 794 *CPM* Chap. 24. *GP* pp. 538–47.

5. b) is appropriate.

One must be willing to take more initiative in developing the relationship which is the central therapeutic modality. The other suggestions can be dangerous. A passive response is risky and ineffective; there should be an early focus on symptom relief, and the involvement of personal resources may be crucial.

Hatton C. L. *et al.* (1977).
CTP Chap. 27.1 pp. 704–10 *CPM* Chap. 28 pp. 556–61. *GP* pp. 425–6, 434–7.

6. e)

Though further studies are needed, it appears that at least low levels of chlordiazepoxide, amitriptyline, imipramine, haloperidol, phenothiazines, mono-amine-oxidase inhibitors and chlorazepate are excreted in breast milk. Diazepam and its metabolites are similarly excreted, and maternal doses of diazepam may cause weight loss and lethargy in nursing infants. Meprobamate should certainly be avoided as it is not merely excreted but concentrated in the breast milk at concentrations two to four times the plasma level.

Anderson P. O. (1979); Ayd F. J. (1973); Erkkola R., Kanta J. (1972); Patrick M. T., *et al.* (1972).

7. Postoperative psychiatric problems are seen in what proportion of renal transplant patients?
   a) 0.5%
   b) 2%
   c) 8%
   d) 32%
   e) 65%

8. Which of the following are features typical of the borderline syndrome?
   a) Consistent blandness of effect
   b) High self-esteem
   c) Primitive idealization
   d) Impulsive behaviour
   e) Splitting

9. With regard to the field of consultation–liaison psychiatry, which of these statements is/are true?
   a) Pre-operative psychotherapy or counselling has not been shown to reduce psychological effects of heart surgery
   b) Denial is undesirable and should be discouraged
   c) In surgery for low back pain, psychological factors may be good predictors of functional improvement from surgery
   d) In cardiovascular surgery, mild pre-operative anxiety is generally associated with good outcome
   e) There are significant differences between rates of postoperative psychological complications in coronary bypass surgery and in heart valve surgery

Answers overleaf

7. d)

Around one-third show psychiatric problems, commonly depression and anxiety; over 10% show an organic brain syndrome.

Strain J. J., Grossman S. (1975).
GP pp. 138–40.

8. c), d), e)

a) No, *intense* effect, often hostile or depressive, inconsistent and variable, is typical.

b) No, low self-esteem is typical, with feelings of emptiness and inadequacy.

c) Yes, similar to splitting, this is a tendency to view external objects as either wholly good or wholly bad, by criteria derived from the patient's own idiosyncratic needs, creating unrealistic expectations.

d) Yes, poor impulse control, as well as episodic acts of self-mutilation and acting out, are typical.

e) Yes, splitting is a psychological defense, showing a division of self and external objects into all good and all bad categories, and can show sudden reversals of categorization.

Kernberg O. F. (1975); Mack J. E. (1975).
CTP Chap. 20 pp. 487–90. *GP* p. 269.

9. c), d), e)

a) No, this does produce significantly lower rates of postoperative delirium.

b) No, denial is extremely valuable, and should rarely be interfered with; only in extremes, when it is preventing essential treatment, is modification needed.

c) Yes, for example, hypochondriasis and hysteria scales on the MMPI predict surgery results, high scores suggesting poor results.

d) Yes, though severe anxiety and depression are associated with greater morbidity and mortality.

e) Yes, the rates are lower after coronary bypass surgery.

Strain J. J., Grossman S. (1975).

10. Which of these symptoms are NOT typical of post-traumatic stress disorders?
   a) Flashbacks
   b) Guilt
   c) Difficulty with interpersonal closeness
   d) Irritability
   e) Euphoria

11. Causes of potentially reversible organic brain syndrome in the elderly include:
   a) Trauma
   b) Reactions to medication
   c) Infection
   d) Alzheimer's disease
   e) Atherosclerosis

12. In the fetal alcohol syndrome:
   a) It only occurs with alcohol intake above 8 ounces (15–20 drinks) a day
   b) There is usually mild or moderate mental retardation
   c) There is usually a high birth weight
   d) Facial abnormalities occur significantly often
   e) Liver abnormalities occur significantly often

Answers overleaf

10. e)

Only euphoria, of the options listed, is not typical of post-traumatic stress disorders which are related to what has also been called combat neurosis or shell-shock.

Figley C. R. (1978).
CTP Chap. 19.4, pp. 446-51.

11. a), b), c)

a) Yes, especially subdural hematoma in those prone to falls.
b) Yes. The elderly use twice as much prescription medication as the young, while impaired metabolism and increased sensitivity of drug receptor sites increase risk of adverse side effects.
c) Yes. Decline in immunocompetence with age predisposes to infections, while classical signs and symptoms may be absent or less clear and intense than usual in the elderly.
d) and e) No, these are irreversible processes.

CTP Chap. 18, pp. 386-425. *GP* pp. 69-127, 326, 403-5.

12. b), d)

a) No. Even 2 ounces (4 or 5 drinks) a day can produce a 12% rate of FAS.
b) Yes, it is now believed to be a common cause of mental retardation.
c) No, there is a low initial birth weight and length.
d) Yes, anomalous epicanthal folds, ptosis, cleft lip and palate, maxillary hypoplasia, and others occur.
e) No, though renal deficits, including hydronephrosis and small rotated kidneys, do occur.

CTP pp. 531-2. *CPM* Chap. 12-6.

13. Milieu therapy:

a) Uses the interaction between the patient and the social environment to produce therapeutic change
b) Was originally described by Pierre Milieu
c) Has been notably developed by Maxwell Jones
d) Uses concepts only applicable in certain special units
e) Uses concepts derived from systems theory

14. An example of *primary* prevention of mental illness would be:

a) Crisis intervention
b) Providing parents with training in child-rearing
c) Vocational rehabilitation programmes
d) Partial hospitalization
e) Alcoholics Anonymous

15. Benzodiazepines with a short half-life include:

a) Lorazepam
b) Clorazepate
c) Diazepam
d) Oxazepam
e) Geripram

Answers overleaf

13. a), c), e)

a) Yes.
b) No, there was no such person. 'Milieu' is environment.
c) Yes, see reference.
d) No, most of its concepts apply to almost any therapeutic setting.
e) Yes, amongst its rather eclectic bases.

Jones M. (1953); Rapaport R. N. (1967).
CTP pp. 333–4 *GP* p. 373.

14. b)

Primary prevention strives to eliminate factors causing or contributing to the development of disease, rather than to deal with already extant disease or problems. Rehabilitation and AA are examples of *tertiary* prevention, an effort to reduce residual disability after an illness of treatment.

CPM pp. 546–7.

15. a), d)

Lorazepam and oxazepam have a short half-life (8–20 hours); diazepam and clorazepate have long half-lives (44 hours or more). Geripram does not exist.

CTP Chap. 29.3, pp. 812–5 *CPM* pp. 488–91 *GP* pp. 533–5.

16. Briquet's syndrome is:

a) Related to heavy alcohol consumption
b) Also known as somatization disorder
c) Characterized by recurrent multiple somatic complaints with no organic basis
d) Usually treated successfully with surgery
e) Characterized by features of multiple personality

17. Using Antabuse/disulfiram in treating alcoholism:

a) The drug acts by blocking the metabolism of paraldehyde
b) There are no noticeable effects from normal doses, unless alcohol is consumed
c) At least 10 days must elapse from the last dose before one might drink without a toxic reaction
d) Usual dose is around 500 mg for 5 days, and 250 mg a day thereafter
e) Toxic reactions include sweating, palpitations, flushing, nausea and vomiting

18. In phenylketonuria:

a) It is transmitted as a sex-linked recessive trait
b) The patient is unable to convert paratyrosine to phenylalanine
c) There is an abnormal metabolite, phenylpyruvic acid, in the urine
d) There is absence or inactivity of the enzyme phenylalanine hydroxylase
e) Abnormal EEG findings are rare

Answers overleaf

16. b), c)

a) No, there is no such relation.

d) No, quite the contrary.

e) No, multiple personality is a very rare disorder, almost always complicated by the therapist's over-involvement and encouragement of the development of new personalities and picturesque features. It is a syndrome of joint pathology, of therapist and patient.

CTP Chap. 19.5, pp. 451–3, 465–6 *CPM* pp. 383–4 *GP* p. 203.

17. d), e)

a) No, it blocks the metabolism of acetaldehyde.

b) No, there may be drowsiness, fatigue, dizziness, skin rash or an odd metallic taste, though these may be avoidable by reducing the dosage.

c) No, usually 2 to 5 days must elapse.

d) Yes.

e) Yes, as well as dyspnea, hypotension and drowsiness.

CTP pp. 409–10, 536–7 *CPM* pp. 205–6 *GP* pp. 215–6.

18. c), d)

a) No, it is transmitted as a simple recessive autosomal Mendelian trait.

b) No, the patient cannot convert phenylalanine to paratyrosine.

c) Yes, there is excess phenylpyruvic acid as well as excess phenylalanine.

d) Yes, this is central to the metabolic anomaly.

e) No, the EEG findings are abnormal in about 80% of patients, even when there are no convulsions.

Robinson G. B., Robinson N. M. (1975); Stanbury J. B. *et al.*, (1972). *CTP* p. 853 *CPM* p. 405 *GP* pp. 444–6.

19. The most commonly observed EEG sleep anomalies in primary depressive disorders are:
   a) Decreased REM and n-REM activity
   b) Increased REM and decreased n-REM activity
   c) Increased REM activity and decreased REM latency
   d) Increased REM activity and increased REM latency
   e) Decreased REM and increased n-REM activity

20. Administration of benzodiazepines results in:
   a) Binding of gamma–amino–butyric acid (GABA)
   b) Mobilizing of chloride ions
   c) Binding of monoamine oxidase (MAO)
   d) Binding of noradrenaline (norepinephrine)
   e) Binding of chloride ions

21. In patients with neurotic disorders, comparing results of therapy with spontaneous improvement rates in untreated patients:
   a) All forms of psychotherapy are less effective
   b) Only psychoanalysis is more effective
   c) All forms of orthodox psychotherapy are more effective
   d) Only behaviour therapy is more effective
   e) Only group therapy is more effective

Answers overleaf

19. c)

Increased REM activity and decreased REM latency is commonly seen in primary depression.

Kupfer D. J. *et al.* (1980).
CPM pp. 51–2. *GP* pp. 325–6.

20. a), b)

Paul S. M. (1981).
GP pp. 533–5.

21. c)

The weight of evidence suggests that all regular forms of psychotherapy yield significantly better results than the so-called spontaneous improvement rate (improvement while remaining untreated during a period equivalent to that of therapy). No one form of intervention is consistently better than another for all forms of problems.

Luborsky L., Singer B., Luborsky L. (1976).
CTP, Chap. 28 *CPM* Chap. 25 pp. 502. *GP* pp. 336, 593, 595–6.

22. Which of the following statements are NOT true about Phencyclidine (PCP)?

a) The best management of PCP intoxication is simply to 'talk down' a patient
b) PCP shows depressant, stimulant and hallucinogen-like effects
c) Specific PCP binding sites have been identified in rat brain membranes
d) Other drugs can interact with the PCP receptor and compete for binding
e) Enkephalins can interact with the PCP receptor, and compete for binding

23. Substances believed to have actions in the brain, relevant in memory function, include:

a) Vasopressin
b) Serotonin
c) Somatostatin
d) LH-RH
e) TRH

24. The animus, in Jungian thought, is defined as:

a) Masculine contrasexual elements in women
b) Feminine contrasexual elements in men
c) The equivalent of the Freudian concept of libido
d) Repressed sexual impulses
e) Repressed hostility

Answers overleaf

22. a), e)

PCP shows mixed effects and may produce coma, convulsions, delirium, acute hypertension, later depression, schizophreniform psychosis, aggressiveness, unexpected muscular strength, impulsivity, hypoalgesia, and rage, and the patient may show vertical nystagmus. Specific PCP receptor sites have been demonstrated in the CNS, and bound PCP can only be displaced by drugs which show PCP-like effects in animal behavioural tests. Drugs which can interact with the PCP receptor, and displace it, include ketamine, cyclohexamine, cyclazocine and pentazocine. Other opiates, morphine, naloxone, enkephalins and endorphin do *not* do so. These findings suggest that a PCP antagonist might be synthesized. (a) and (e) are not true, and hence the correct answers. (b), (c) and (d) are true.

Showalter C. V., Thornton W. E. (1977); Zukin S. R., Zukin R. S. (1979).
CTP pp. 521–3. *CPM* p. 219. *GP* pp. 232, 235–6.

23. a)

Vasopressin, a peptide hormone, in addition to its renal, antidiuretic effects, has actions in the brain including maintenance and enhancement of memory and other cognitive functions, and may be relevant to the biochemistry of depression.

Schlesser M. A. *et al.* (1980).
CPM pp. 46–7.

24. a)

(a) Correctly defines the animus; (b) describes the anima; the other responses are wrong.

Jung C. G. (1966).
CTP Chap. 8.3 pp. 160–1. *CPM* pp. 22–3. *GP* pp. 30–1.

25. Which of the following treatments have been clearly shown to be effective in reversing memory problems due to senile dementia in the elderly?

  a) Hyperbaric oxygen
  b) Vasodilators
  c) Lecithin
  d) Anticoagulants
  e) None of the above

26. Features common to all forms of psychotherapy include all of the following EXCEPT:

  a) A rational or conceptual scheme that explains the cause of the patient's difficulties and prescribes a way to combat them, convincing to both participants
  b) A trusting, confiding, emotionally active relationship between a patient seeking help and a therapist offering it
  c) A setting clearly distinguished from daily life
  d) The therapist's attitude of acceptance and respect for the patients, not necessarily for what they are, but for what they could become
  e) An emphasis on the continuing relevance and exploration of early childhood experiences

27. Which of the common side-effects of lithium carbonate may be MORE common with slow-release preparations?

  a) Nausea
  b) Tremor
  c) Thirst
  d) Diarrhoea
  e) None of the above

Answers overleaf

25. e)

None of these treatments have been convincingly found to have reliably useful effects in this situation.

Birren J., Sloan R. R. (1980); Busse E., Blazer D. (1980).
CTP p. 395. *CPM* p. 281.

26. e) is not a common feature, and is used in only some of the many psychotherapies, while (a), (b), (c) and (d) do describe features common to all psychotherapies.

Luborsky L., Singer B., Luborsky L. (1976).
CTP Chap. 28. *CPM* Chap. 25. *GP* pp. 561–600.

27. d)

Most symptoms (such as (a) (b) and (c)), are related to the higher peak blood levels following absorption. Slow-release preparations reduce these problems. But excessive unabsorbed lithium may, with slow release forms, reach the lower intestine and can lead to a higher incidence of diarrhoea..

Jefferson J. W., Griest J. H. (1972).
CTP, p. 406, Chap. 29.7 pp. 825–9. *CPM* pp. 455–457. *GP* pp. 550–1.

28. The characteristics of near-death experiences are:
   a) Exclusively seen in life-threatening situations
   b) Not related to other forms of out-of-the-body experience
   c) Seen in other altered states of consciousness
   d) Were first described by R. Moody
   e) Are evidence of the existence of life after death

29. Spontaneous panic attacks (in the absence of other significant psychiatric symptoms) generally respond best to:
   a) Chlorpromazine
   b) Chlorimipramine
   c) MAO Inhibitors
   d) Diazepam
   e) Alcohol

30. Which of the following major figures have NOT been noted for their contributions to the understanding of the borderline syndrome and borderline personality disorder?
   a) Roy Grinker
   b) Carl Rogers
   c) Otto Kernberg
   d) Hans Kohut
   e) Helen Singer Kaplan

Answers overleaf

28. c)

The features of the NDA are commonly seen in other varieties of altered states, so (a) and (b) are wrong; (d) is also wrong. Although Moody received a great deal of publicity, he was very far from the first person to describe a phenomenon recognized for centuries; (e) is wrong, as they occur during life, not after death.

Noyes R. (1979); Stevenson I., Greyson B. (1979).

29. b), c)

The efficacy of chlorpromazine and MAO inhibitors have been shown in numerous clinical studies. Benzodiazepines seem more effective with anticipatory anxiety and worrisome expectation; beta-blockers can deal with the accompanying autonomic overactivity.

CTP Chap. 19.1 pp. 426–31. *CPM* p. 395.

30. b), e)

a), c) and d) have made major contributions to the understanding of this important clinical entity, much neglected and misunderstood in Britain. Grinker and his associates helped delineate the characteristics of the syndrome; Kernberg described its psychodynamics, as did Kohut. Carl Rogers has made many great contributions, including client-centred therapy; and Helen Kaplan is noted for her work in sex therapy, but neither has worked on the borderline syndrome. Other major contributors to this field have been Gunderson and Masterson.

Grinker R. R. *et al.* (1968); Kernberg O. F. (1975); Kohut H. (1971). *CTP* Chap. 20, pp. 487–90.

31. Which of the following characteristics is/are typical of encounter groups?
   a) Carefully planned and specified agenda or tasks
   b) Exercises deliberately aimed at exploring childhood dynamics
   c) A closely defined leadership structure within the group
   d) A free environment in which task and structure are supplied by the members themselves
   e) All of the above

32. If you consider that there are strong grounds to continue lithium maintenance therapy during a particular pregnant patient's therapy, apart from trying to ascertain the lowest serum level which will maintain a euthymic state in this person, which of the following are true statements, relevant in forming your plans?
   a) Lithium retention increases shortly after delivery
   b) Lithium is excreted in breast milk
   c) Maternal lithium clearance often increases substantially during pregnancy
   d) All of the above
   e) None of the above

33. Signs of damage to the posterior columns include:
   a) Loss of deep pain sensation
   b) Ataxia with the eyes open, but not with the eyes closed
   c) Brisk tendon reflexes
   d) Hypotonicity
   e) Loss of proprioception and vibration sense

Answers overleaf

31. d)

The encounter group does not use a specified agenda, tasks, exercises, leadership structure or roles. Members must supply these elements for themselves and, in the process, must deal on the basis of their own needs and resources with problems of power, influence and decision-making.

Bion W. H. (1959); Lieberman M. A. *et al*. (1973; Rogers C. (1970).
CTP pp. 758, 726.

32. d)

All the statements are true. Lithium is excreted in breast milk at concentrations about half of those in the mother's serum. The most frequently occurring congenital abnormalities in offspring of women who take lithium during the first trimester of pregnancy involve cardiovascular malformations.

Jefferson J. W., Griest J. H. (1972).
CTP Chap. 29.7, pp. 825-9. *CPM* pp. 451-69. *GP* p. 553.

33. a), d), e)

Signs of posterior column damage include: loss of deep pain sensation (a), with positive Rombergism (the opposite of statement (b)) as the lack of proprioception can be corrected for by looking at the position of the limbs; (c) is wrong—there are diminished tendon reflexes. The sensory stimulus for the deep reflexes is a stretch (and hence proprioceptive) reflex, diminished by the reduction in proprioception; (d) is correct—there is hypotonicity, as many spinocerebellar fibres travel in the posterior columns before entering the spinocerebellar tract; (e) is right, as proprioception and vibration sense are carried via the posterior columns.

Walton J. N. (1977).
CTP Chap. 2.2 pp. 33-45.

34. Which of the following is the most strongly anticholinergic antidepressants?

   a) Amitriptyline
   b) Desipramine
   c) Protriptyline
   d) Phenelzine
   e) Thiothixine

35. You ask a patient to explain the meaning of the proverb: 'People who live in glass houses shouldn't throw stones'. He replies: 'They'd break the windows—or is this about solar energy?'
The response can best be described as:

   a) Irrelevant
   b) Illogical
   c) Concrete
   d) Stupid
   e) Circumstantial

36. In the syndrome of minimal brain dysfunction (MBD)

   a) Children show no sign of altered CNS functioning
   b) Increase in motor activity is due to anxiety
   c) Hyperactivity may respond to psychostimulant drugs
   d) Medication, if effective, will need to be used life-long
   e) Learning disabilities may include problems in processing sensory input

Answers overleaf

34. a)

Amitriptyline is the most strongly anticholinergic. Thiothixine is not an antidepressant, but an antipsychotic.

CTP Chap. 29.2, pp. 789–97. *CPM* pp. 443–45, 448–51. *GP* pp. 517, 538–45.

35. c)

This is a concrete response, possibly indicative of psychopathology. The other descriptors are inaccurate and unhelpful.

CTP Chap. 10, pp. 194–195. *CPM* p. 168. *GP* p. 353.

36. c), e)

a) No, about 40% show such signs, including learning disabilities, hyperactivity, distractibility and short attention span.

b) No, hyperactivity is physiologically based, not caused by anxiety, may be present from birth, and is not situationally responsive to peaceful or anxiety-provoking situations.

c) Yes, most commonly used medications include: dextroamphetamine, methylphenidate and pemoline.

d) No, some seem not to need it after 13 to 15 years of age; perhaps 15% need to continue medication through adolescence and into young adulthood. It is not generally considered necessary beyond that.

e) Yes, perception may be disturbed, as may cognition and memory.

Cantwell D. (1975); Wender P. H. (1971).
CTP Chap. 34 pp. 875–83. *CPM* pp. 318–19. *GP* pp. 488–90.

37. Characteristic features of upper motor neurone lesions include:
   a) Anti-gravity muscles are affected most
   b) Clasp-knife rigidity
   c) Loss of muscle bulk
   d) Decreased deep tendon reflexes
   e) Extensor plantor responses

38. Drugs which may be useful in the treatment of *pavor nocturnus* (night terrors) and somnambulism include:
   a) Amphetamines
   b) Chloral hydrate
   c) Flurazepam
   d) Diazepam
   e) Frusemide

39. In follow-up studies of chronic schizophrenic patients, which characteristic(s) observed at the time of initial evaluation emerge as predictors of 5-year outcome?
   a) Work function
   b) Thought disorder
   c) Level of social contact
   d) Duration of previous hospitalization
   e) Positive family history of schizophrenia

Answers overleaf

37. a), b), e)

a) Yes, anti-gravity muscles, like flexors of the arms and extensors of the legs, are most affected.
b) Yes, clasp-knife rigidity, with initially increased resistance to extension of the affected limb and then marked loss of resistance, is characteristic.
c) No, bulk tends to be preserved, modified only by secondary disuse atrophy. Loss of bulk is more typical of lower motor neurone lesions.
d) No, they are increased, often with clonus; decrease of tendon reflexes is typical of lower motor neurone lesions.
e) Yes.

38. b), c), d)

Sedative drugs which suppress stage 4 sleep and do not suppress REM sleep, are useful in *pavor nocturnus* and somnambulism.

CTP p. 682.

39. a), c), d)

Duration of previous hospitalization, level of functioning social contact and work function have been found to be good predictors of outcome at 5 years; family history of schizophrenia and presence of active thought disorder were not predictors of outcome.

Strauss J. S., Carpenter W. T. (1977).

GP pp. 376–7.

40. Compared to heroin, withdrawal from methadone is usually:
a) More rapid
b) More gradual
c) More dangerous
d) More likely to precipitate psychosis
e) More likely to produce severe symptoms

41. Prospective and double-blind controlled studies have suggested that predictors of good response to tricyclic antidepressants include:
a) Anorexia and weight loss
b) Lower socioeconomic class
c) Middle and late insomnia
d) Psychomotor retardation
e) Multiple prior episodes

42. Which of the following statements about sexuality and disability are true?
a) Sexual dysfunction is rare in dialysis patients
b) About 25% of paraplegic males can have reflex erections which will allow intercourse
c) Organic impotence occurs in diabetic men
d) Acute or chronic use of alcohol can cause erectile dysfunction
e) Alcohol is rarely a cause of ejaculatory difficulties

Answers overleaf

40. b)

Withdrawal from methadone is usually more gradual than withdrawal from heroin.

Gilman A., Goodman L. S., Gilman A. (1980).
CTP p. 509. *GP* pp. 224–5.

41. a), c), d)

b) Not true—the upper socioeconomic class tends to respond better; and e) is not true, as people with multiple prior episodes are poor responders.

Bielsk R. J., Friedel R. O. (1976).

42. b), c), d)

a) No, many dialysis patients report sexual dysfunction, due to psychological and biological factors, including depression, stresses of chronic illness, and biochemical and endocrine disturbances.

b) Yes, several studies have shown that around 50% of men with spinal cord injuries can get erections in response to genital stimulation. In about half of these, the quality and duration was sufficient to allow intercourse. Orgasm and ejaculation are rare, however.

c) Yes, impotence, due to neuropathic changes, major vessel obstructions and microangiopathies is relatively common. Therapy may be effective in some cases.

d) Yes, many men experience one or more episodes of erectile failure due to alcohol, and this is more common with chronic alcohol use.

e) No, alcohol commonly causes delayed ejaculation, probably more commmonly than any other cause.

GP pp. 252–3.

43. Regarding optimal management of severe tricyclic antidepressant poisoning, which of the following statements is true?

a) Gastric aspiration and lavage is of no value beyond 6 hours after ingestion of the drug
b) Cardiorespiratory support and cardiac monitoring is important
c) Anti-arrhythmic drugs should be used routinely
d) Convulsions may occur and need prompt treatment
e) Physostigmine may reverse some of the symptoms

44. A young patient describes experiencing diplopia in the afternoons and occasional difficulty chewing and swallowing her evening meal. Which of the following procedures is most likely to help confirm the correct diagnosis?

a) CT scan
b) Electromyography
c) Exercise tolerance tests
d) The 'Tensilon test', administering edrophonium
e) Tomography of the mediastinum

45. In Piaget's classification, pre-operational thinking

a) is a feature of children 2 to 6 years old
b) is a feature of children 1 to 2 years of age
c) includes egocentricity
d) includes abstraction
e) includes animism

Answers overleaf

43. b), d), e)

a) No, TCAs delay gastric emptying and the tablets may remain in the stomach longer than usual. Gastric lavage may be useful for up to 12 hours after the ingestion of the overdose.

b) Yes, TCA overdose decreases myocardial contractility and increases conduction times; and a variety of arrhythmias may occur, including sinus bradycardia, supraventricular and ventricular tachycardias, ventricular fibrillation and sinus rhythm with grossly prolonged atrioventricular and intraventricular condition times.

c) No, though this seems appropriate, such drugs are not needed in a majority of cases, and the tachycardias which occur are of less serious significance than when they occur after a myocardial infarction, according to some authorities. More important, some drugs such as disopyramide, lignocaine and β-adrenergic blockers can *potentiate* tricyclic—induced cardiotoxicity.

d) Yes, intravenous diazepam and chlormethiazole are probably the agents of choice. As these drugs may further depress respiration, they should be used with caution.

e) Yes, intravenous physostigmine salicylate, a cholinesterase inhibitor which crosses the blood-brain barrier, can reverse some symptoms including delirium, coma, choreo-athetosis and tremor. Unfortunately it has risks itself if too large a dose is injected, and it has a short duration of action (usually less than 45 minutes).

CTP pp. 795–7. *GP* 542.

44. d)

The symptoms are typical of myasthenia gravis. Edrophonium/Tensilon is a very short-acting anticholinesterase agent and produces a temporary increase in strength in this condition, and reversal of symptoms.

GP p. 131.

45. a), c), e)

Pre-operational thinking, according to Piaget, occurs in children from about 2 to 6 years of age. They respond egocentrically to perceptions rather than using abstract concepts. They do not yet recognize the reversibility of operations, and tend to endow inanimate objects with animate qualities (animism).

Piaget (1929, 1952); Flavell (1963)
CTP Chap. 3.2 pp. 55–9. *CPM* pp. 401–402, 605–6. *GP* 464–5.

46. It has been proposed that tardive dyskinesia may be related to an underlying dopaminergic–cholinergic imbalance, because:
   a) Sympathomimetics may make the syndrome worse
   b) Choline fails to relieve symptoms
   c) Dopamine blockers (like antipsychotic drugs) can alleviate the syndrome for a short time
   d) L-dopa can produce similar movement disorders when taken in excess
   e) All of the above

47. In Carl Rogers' work, the central components of the process of psychotherapy are:
   a) Empathy
   b) Reflection of the patient's feelings
   c) Unconditional positive regard for the patient
   d) Interpretation of the transference relationship
   e) Explanation of unconscious processes

48. Formication
   a) is an alternative term for extra-marital sex
   b) is a variety of hallucination of touch
   c) may occur in cocaine psychosis
   d) is uncommon in delirium
   e) is the sensation of insects crawling over the body

Answers overleaf

46. a), c), d)

e) and b) are incorrect. Choline can relieve the symptoms in a proportion of cases (though it may produce a serious side-effect of psychotic depression).

   a) True—sympathomimetics (which release dopamine) may worsen the syndrome.
   c) True. Dopamine blockers like antipsychotic drugs can alleviate the symptoms for a time, though the body may adapt by adding new receptors.
   d) True.

CTP pp. 265, 785. *CPM* pp. 480–4. *GP* pp. 531–3.

47. a), b), c)

Carl Rogers' view of client-centred therapy stresses the importance of empathic understanding, unconditional positive regard for the client, and reflection of feelings. It does not use interpretation of unconscious or transference issues.

Rogers C (1970).
CTP Chap. 28.6 pp. 764–6. *GP* p. 599.

48. b), c), e)

   a) No, that would be fornication.
   b) Yes, it not uncommon in acute brain syndromes.
   c) Yes, sometimes known as the 'cocaine bug'.
   d) No, it is relatively common in delirium.
   e) Yes, that is its definition.

49. The following benzodiazepines have active metabolities:
   a) Diazepam
   b) Chlordiazepoxide
   c) Oxazepam
   d) Lorazepam
   e) Clorazepate

50. A 55-year-old man complains of decreased libido and erectile impotence for a year. Steps to help decide whether these complaints have an organic or functional basis should include:
   a) Interview his sexual partner separately
   b) Ask the patient about nocturnal tumescence
   c) Laboratory tests are not indicated and unlikely to be helpful
   d) A history of drug use is usually non-contributory
   e) A history of alcohol use is helpful

51. Pseudohallucinations may occur in:
   a) Hysteria
   b) Borderline syndrome
   c) Hypnogogic states
   d) Phobic anxiety state
   e) Bereavement

Answers overleaf

49. a), b), e)

Diazepam has active metabolites (N-desmethyldiazepam/oxazepam), as does chlordiazepoxide (N-desmethylchlordiazepoxide/demoxepam and N-desmethyldiazepam/oxazepam) and clorazepate (also oxazepam). Oxazepam itself and lorazepam do not have active metabolites. As a result, the half lives differ—12 to 20 hours for oxazepam, 12 hours for lorazepam, 26–35 hours for diazepam, and 8–28 hours for chlordiazepoxide.

CTP Chap. 29.3, pp. 802–5. *CPM* pp. 489–91. *GP* pp. 533–5.

50. a), b), e)

a) Yes, her version may differ from his and provide extra insights into the problem, and one should avoid involving only one partner in the management of a sexual problem.

b) Yes, the occurrence of nocturnal tumescence shows the integrity of the reflex arc.

c) No, a glucose tolerance test may be useful. It is estimated that some 50% of diabetics show impotence in their 50s. A serum testosterone level could help identify low androgen levels as a cause of impotence.

d) No, antihypertensives, tranquillizers and drugs with anticholinergic effects (including tricyclic antidepressants, and antiparkinsonian agents) may affect libido and erectile facility.

e) Yes, alcohol may also effect libido and erectile facility.

Masters W. H., Johnson V. E. (1970); Kaplan H. S. (1974).
CTP Chap. 22.4 pp. 561–8, Chap. 22.5 pp. 568–70. *GP*, pp. 252–3.

51. a), c), e)

Pseudohallucinations are vivid sensory experiences based on internal rather than external events, in the absence of an external stimulus. But, unlike hallucinations, the person recognizes them as unreal. They can occur in hysterical pseudopsychosis, hypnogogic and hypnopompic states (while drifting into and out of sleep); in bereavement, fatigue, trance, sensory and sleep deprivation, and may occur with some psychotomimetic drugs. They are usually auditory or visual.

CPM p. 567.

52. Patients with delirium:

a) Experience visual hallucinations
b) Are best nursed in a darkened room
c) Are rarely disoriented for time
d) Experience illusions
e) Are best sedated with barbiturates

53. You forget a patient's appointment and make arrangements for another meeting at the same time. You should:

a) Blame the mistake on your secretary or receptionist
b) Offer a dynamic interpretation of the patient's feelings of anger and rejection
c) Recognize this may be an instance of countertransference and explore this possibility by introspection
d) Squeeze in an extra appointment for the patient after the rest of your appointments that day
e) Avoid making a personal apology lest it be misinterpreted by the patient

54. Which of the following agents are used as psychotomimetic inhalants by substance abusers?

a) Neon
b) Freon
c) Myristicin
d) Toluene
e) Acetone

Answers overleaf

52. a), d)

Patients with delirium are usually disoriented for time and space, and are best nursed in a light room with as many visual clues as possible to aid maintenance of orientation. They experience visual hallucinations and illusions; but they should not be sedated with drugs such as barbiturates which can compound the delirium and confusion.

CTP Chap. 18, pp. 386-91. *CPM* Chap. 12, pp. 266-73.

53. c) is an appropriate response.

a), b), d) and e) are rude and unhelpful.

Singer E. (1970).
CTP pp. 177-8, 730. *GP* p. 566.

54. b), d), e)

a) No. Neon is an inert gas.

b) Yes. Freon is used as a psychotomimetic inhalant, as is (d) toluene and (e) acetone—as well as model aeroplane glue, paint thinners, petrol/kerosene and other aerosols.

c) Myristicin is a psychotomimetic (a component of nutmeg) but not an inhalant.

CPM p. 218. *GP* p. 231.

55. Characteristic features of psychotic depression include:

a) *Deja vu*
b) Racing thoughts
c) Delusions of sin or guilt
d) Visual hallucinations
e) Nihilism

56. With regard to benzodiazepines, it is generally well-documented that:

a) Benodiazepine-specific receptors have been found in the brain
b) Clinical potency of benzodiazepines correlates with their affinity for these receptors
c) Their actions involve the neurotransmitter gamma-aminobutyric acid (GABA)
d) Their actions definitely involve dopamine synthesis
e) Their actions definitely involve serotonin depletion

57. Which of the following statements about child abuse are NOT true?

a) Prematurely born children are more likely to be abused than full term children
b) Parents who abuse children were often abused when they themselves were children
c) Parents are more likely to abuse one child than to abuse all of their children
d) Fathers are more likely to abuse the children than mothers
e) Older children are more often abused than younger children

Answers overleaf

55. c), e)

Psychotic depression characteristically features depressive delusions with themes of guilt, sin, nihilism, worthlessness, poverty, illness and doom. *Deja vu*, racing thoughts and visual hallucinations are not found.

CTP p. 361. *GP* p. 329.

56. a), b), c)

Benzodiazepine receptors have been recently discovered and are not involved in the action of other sedative hypnotics. Researchers are looking for an endogenous ligand for these receptors, analogous to the endorphins. The effects of GABA seem relevant to the sedative actions of benzodiazepines, and also to their muscle relaxant and anticonvulsant effects. There are some data on benzodiazepine effects on other neurotransmitters—dopamine, serotonin, and noradrenaline (norepinephrine), but the implications are not clear.

57. d), e)

Mothers abuse their children more often than fathers, and children under the age of 3 years are more often affected. Parents who abuse children are often people who were abused by their own parents. Individual children seem to become 'scapegoats', singled out for abuse—they are more often prematurely born and slower to develop than their siblings.

GP pp. 490–1.

58. Among the activation techniques used in electroencephalograpy is/are:

a) Photic stimulation
b) Anticonvulsant drugs
c) Sleep
d) Hyperventilation
e) All of the above

59. All of the following statements about Down's Syndrome are true, EXCEPT:

a) It is often due to an extra chromasome in Group G
b) It is often caused by nondysfunction during meiosis of the oocyte
c) Nondysfunction occurs during meiosis of the sperm
d) It may be due to chromosomal translocation
e) All of the above

60. Which of these are NOT among Schneider's first-rank symptoms?

a) Thought insertion
b) Feelings of passivity
c) Secondary delusions
d) Voices talking about the patient in the third person
e) Clouding of consciousness

Answers overleaf

58. a), c), d)

Activation techniques include sleep, photic stimulation, over-breathing, and, more rarely, overhydration or alcohol.

GP p. 110.

59. c), e)

a) Yes, in around 90% of instances there is an extra small acrocentric chromosome in group G, giving trisomy 21, and 47 rather than 46 chromosomes.
b) Yes.
c) No, there is faulty meiosis of the oocyte.
d) Yes, this is less commonly the cause than (a), but more often the case when a young mother has produced a child with Down's syndrome (mongolism).
e) No.

CTP pp. 859–60. *CPM* pp. 403–4. *GP* pp. 449–52.

60. c), e)

a) Yes, also thought withdrawal and thought broadcast.
b) Yes, experiencing sensations, emotions or movement as being caused by, or controlled by, some outside agency.
c) No, *primary* delusions—the sudden appearance of fully formed delusions from a normal perception are first rank features. Secondary delusions, arising from and explaining other symptoms like hallucinations, are not.
d) Yes.
e) No. In fact clear consciousness is important in diagnosing schizophrenia. Clouding of consciousness suggests organic impairment and casts doubts on the diagnosis.

CTP p. 295. *GP* pp. 357–8.

61. Benzodiazepines concentrate in:

a) The limbic system
b) The frontal cortex
c) The thalamic nuclei
d) The reticular formation
e) The cerebellum

62. A 40-year-old previously emotionally healthy pre-menopausal woman recently underwent an abdominal hysterectomy with conservation of the ovaries, for dysfunctional uterine bleeding. Now she complains of loss of libido, and finds her husband's sexual advances distasteful. Likely causes include:

a) The onset of the menopause
b) Post-hysterectomy psychosis
c) Depression related to feelings of inadequacy as a woman
d) Anxiety related to loss of reproductive capacity
e) Exacerbation of pre-existing sexual dysfunction

63. Investigation of possible intellectual deterioration might usefully include all of the following EXCEPT:

a) Progressive Matrices
b) Mill Hill Vocabulary Scale
c) Bender Gestalt
d) Edwards Personal Preference Schedule (EPPS)
e) Eysenck Personality Inventory

Answers overleaf

61. a), c), d)
Paul S. M. (1981).

62. c), e)

a) No, removal of the uterus does not lead to premature menopause or alter ovarian function. When the ovaries are removed prematurely, depression is around four times more common than in women who have had other comparable surgery.

b) No, hysterectomy does not usually cause psychiatric symptoms postoperatively, except uncommonly in women with significant pre-existing emotional disturbances, in response to aggravation of an already inadequate concept of herself as a woman, and with inadequate support from her husband and doctor.

c) Yes, probably a likely explanation. The hysterectomy may be experienced as a threat to sexual identity, and may affect the husband as well. Counselling of both partners before and after surgery is important.

d) No, probably not a likely cause. Generally nowadays there is less concern specifically about bearing children when over the age of 40, in relation to the more general wish for a smaller family and concerns about the risks to the offspring from a late pregnancy.

e) Yes, pre-existing sexual dysfunction and low libido or distaste for sexuality may be exacerbated after a hysterectomy, which can provide an excuse for stopping activity that has not hitherto been satisfying.

63. d), e)

(a), (b) and (c) are all useful in assessing possible intellectual deterioration; (a) involves increasingly difficult complex pattern completion problems, and b) involves defining standard lists of words of increasing difficulty; (a) is sensitive and (b) relatively resistant to change, enabling one to estimate the degree of deterioration. The Bender Gestalt (c) can identify perceptual disturbances; d) is an attempt to measure psychological needs such as the need for achievement, for order, for autonomy, etc., and (e) is a personality inventory of no use in this instance and of little use in regard to individual cases.

CTP Chap. 10.7 pp. 216–21. *CPM* p. 279. *GP* pp. 9–16.

64. Which of the following statements about sexual dysfunction in marriage are true?

a) Around 50% of normal, well-informed couples report some degree of sexual dysfunction
b) Women's most common dysfunction is the inability to achieve orgasm
c) Women's most common complaints about marital sex are about their partner's timing and means of approach
d) Men's most common reported dysfunction is impotence
e) Sexual dysfunction is commonly related to medically prescribed drugs

65. Skin discoloration and pigment deposits in the eyes have been described in relation to the long-term use of which drug(s)?

a) Thiothixene
b) Thioridazine
c) Haloperidol
d) Chlorpromazine
e) Flupenthixol

66. When ethanol (as in alcoholic drinks) and tricyclic antidepressants (TCA) are taken together, which of the following occurs?

a) Reduction of the sedative effects of ethanol
b) Enhancement of the sedative effects of ethanol
c) Blockage of the depressant effects of ethanol
d) Increase in the cerebral capillary permeability of alcohol
e) No interactive effects

Answers overleaf

64. a), c), e)

a) True. Although 80% of couples, in several surveys, considered their marriages happy and satisfying; 40% of men reported some erectile or ejaculatory dysfunction and 60% of women reported orgasmic or arousal dysfunction; 50% of men and 77% of women described difficulties of lack of interest, inability to relax, etc.

b) Wrong. Difficulty getting aroused at all and difficulty achieving orgasm are reported about equally frequently by about half of married women. About one-third describe difficulties in maintaining excitement.

c) Yes. Women, more often than men, complain that their partner chooses an inconvenient time for intercourse, an inability to relax, being disinterested and 'turned off', and too little foreplay.

d) Wrong. About one-third of men report ejaculating too quickly as a major problem; 16% report problems getting or maintaining an erection, and 4% report delayed ejaculation. Common sexual difficulties described in marriage by men include attraction to a person other than the spouse, disinterest in marital sex, and interest in other than genital sex.

e) Yes, many antihypertensives (e.g. clonidine, methyldopa, reserpine, spironolactone, chlorthalidone, prazosin and hydrochlorothiazide) as well as other drugs, may cause sexual dysfunction.

Masters W. H., Johnson V. E. (1970); Kaplan H. S. (1974).
CTP Chap. 22.4 pp. 561–8. GP pp. 252–3.

65. b), d)

Skin discoloration and pigment deposits in the eye (irregular or stellate opacities in the anterior part of the lens) have been described with long-term use of both thioridazine and chlorpromazine.
CTP p. 788. CPM pp. 485–6.

66. b), d)

Recent research has shown that tricyclic antidepressants induce increase in cerebral capillary permeability, increasing the concentration of ethanol in the brain; in addition to the widely recognized enhancement of sedative effects of the ethanol. That tricyclics can affect the blood-brain barrier is of great potential interest.

67. Urinary MHPG
   a) is a principle metabolite of brain noradrenaline (norepinephrine)
   b) is produced mainly in the adrenals
   c) is of no clinical relevance
   d) is a metabolite of somatostatin
   e) can be measured in a simple bedside test

68. With regard to homicide, a majority of murderers:
   a) Have a history of psychiatric illness
   b) Are friends or relatives of the victim
   c) Have a history of previous psychiatric hospitalization
   d) Have a history of delinquency from an early age
   e) All of the above

69. Which of the following are NOT examples of projective tests?
   a) Sentence Completion Test
   b) Rorschach Test
   c) Thematic Apperception Test (TAT)
   d) Minnesota Multiphasic Personality Inventory (MMPI)
   e) Adjective Check List (ACL)

Answers overleaf

67. a)

Urinary MHPG is a major metabolite of brain noradrenaline (norepinephrine), and of some clinical significance.

Schlesser M. A. *et al.* (1980).

68. b), d)

Most victims are known to their killers, often friends or relatives. As many as 80% of acts of major violence, including murder, are committed by people under the age of 50. People with a previous psychiatric illness or hospitalization are *no* more likely to be homicidal than anyone else.

CPM pp. 561-3. *GP* pp. 326-7, 394-5, 627-9.

69. d), e)

Projective tests are relatively unstructured and have no 'correct' or 'provided' answers. Responses to such tests are assumed to be more responsive to individual characteristics than with more structured tests where the nature of the test itself has more effect on the responses elicited. The Sentence Completion Test, Rorschach and TAT are projective. The MMPI is a structured test with hundreds of items answered 'true', 'false' or 'cannot say'. The ACL is a list of adjectives which may be checked to describe a person..

GP pp. 14-7.

70. Which of the following statements concerning tricyclic antidepressants (TCAs) are true?
   a) There is low binding to plasma protein
   b) Peritoneal and haemodialysis are effective in treating TCA overdose
   c) Tissue levels are 10 times higher than plasma levels
   d) Highest tissue concentration is in fatty tissues
   e) Tissue binding is at 40 to 200 times the plasma levels

71. Which of these statements about mental retardation are true?
   a) There is a family history of mental handicap in over 50% of cases
   b) Subnormality is commoner in urban areas
   c) Subnormality is more common in social class 5 than in social classes 1 and 2
   d) Subnormality is commoner in women
   e) Some 70% of the mentally handicapped can and do live in the community.

72. Characteristic features of lower motor neurone lesions include:
   a) Akathisia
   b) Loss of muscle bulk
   c) Increased deep tendon reflexes
   d) Increased muscle tone
   e) Plantar reflex, if present, is flexor

Answers overleaf

70. c)

a) No, there is *high* binding to plasma protein—85% to 98%. This is why peritoneal and haemodialysis is not effective in overdose of TCA. As haemoperfusion, for example, may have a rate of only 20 L per hour, with only around 2% of the TCA available free and unbound in the plasma, little can be removed. Thus (b) is not true.

c) Yes, but (d) no—highest concentrations occur in myocardial tissue.

e) Yes; small changes in myocardial binding can produce problems of cardiotoxicity.

Calesnick B. (1980).

71. c), e)

a) No, there is a positive family history in only around 17% of cases.

b) No, it is commoner in rural areas.

c) Yes, it is around 9 times more common in social class 5 than in social classes 1 and 2.

d) No, it is commoner in men, by 1.3 to 1.

e) Yes.

GP pp. 439–61.

72. b), e)

a) No, akathisia is not a feature.

b) Yes, loss of muscle bulk may be as great as 50% to 80% in affected muscles, which are flaccid and hypotonic or atonic.

c) No. Reflexes are absent or decreased.

d) No.

e) Yes.

73. In classical Freudian theory, which of these statements are true of the latency stage of development?

   a) Intense sexual curiosity becomes commoner
   b) It occurs under the age of 5 years
   c) It follows resolution of the oedipal complex
   d) It lasts until the genital stage
   e) It involves struggles about toilet training

74. Which of the following comments on the cardiotoxic effects of antipsychotic drugs is/are NOT true?

   a) Their α-adrenergic blocking effects can cause hypotension
   b) Their cholinergic effects can cause tachycardia
   c) The ECG changes they may produce include QRS narrowing
   d) Thioridazine and chlorpromazine are more cardiotoxic than haloperidol
   e) The ECG changes include shortening of the PR and QT intervals

75. Regarding incest, which of these are true statements?

   a) Incest occurs prinicipally among the poor and social class 4
   b) Incest often involves more than one child in a family
   c) Incest does not have lasting effects on the children involved
   d) Mothers quite often know of the occurrence of incest in the family
   e) Incest is usually a one-time incident

Answers overleaf

73. c), d)

The latency stage follows the resolution of the oedipal complex and lasts until the genital stage, so it runs from around 5 to 13 years of age. Sexual curiosity is a more notable feature of the preceding phallic stage and oedipal complex. Struggles about routines, including toilet training, are more typical of the earlier anal phase.

CTP pp. 126–7. *CPM* pp. 22 *GP* p. 22.

74. c), e)

a) True, α-adrenergic blocking effects can cause hypotension.
b) True, cholinergic effects can cause tachycardia.
c) Untrue, as is (e). The ECG changes include QRS widening, due to their quinidine-like activity, and prolongation of PR and QT intervals.
d) True. Generally, low potency antipsychotic agents which thus need higher doses, have greater hypotensive, tachycardiac and other side-effects.

Rosenbaum J. F. (1980).
GP p. 526.

75. b), d)

a) Untrue. Incest occurs at all levels of society.
b) Yes, the first-born daughter is often the first victim with younger daughters subsequently and sequentially involved (sons may also be involved, but this is less common).
c) No, several studies show that incest is related to later problems in the victims including neurotic symptoms and sexual dysfunctions which may last into adult life.
d) Yes, especially in long-standing cases of incest, the mothers not uncommonly know and may tacitly or explicitly support or tolerate father–daughter relationships. In other families, especially when younger children are involved, the mother may only find out later.
e) No, though some instances are single encounters, incest often occurs on frequent occasions over a period of years.

CTP pp. 573–5.

76. A basic technique used in psychoanalysis is:
a) Hypnosis
b) Free association
c) Abreaction
d) Empathy
e) Reinforcement

77. The commonest cause of delirium in the elderly is:
a) Intracranial tumour
b) Cardiovascular disease
c) Over-medication
d) Malnutrition
e) Infections

78. Patients who are well-informed about what to expect during and after surgery (compared to uninformed patients) tend to:
a) Need less analgesia after surgery
b) Have longer stays in hospital after surgery
c) Show less confidence in their surgeon's ability
d) Show less fear just before surgery
e) Show signficantly more emotional disturbances after surgery

Answers overleaf

76. b)

In free association the patients are encouraged to ignore censorship and express all ideas that occur to them. Apart from providing material for analysis, it also serves to help induce the necessary regression while establishing and working through the transference neurosis.

CTP pp. 122, 146–7, 728. GP pp. 562–71.

77. c)

Over-medication is probably the commonest cause of delirium in the elderly; though infections are also common causes, and malnutrition, cardiovascular disease and intracranial tumours are possible but less common causes.

Post F. (1965)
CTP Chap. 42, pp. 1017–22. CPM Chap. 32 pp. 639–53.

78. a)

Well-informed patients need less medication for postoperative pain, are discharged from hospital earlier, are less angry and show more confidence in their surgeons, and recall the operation with less emotional disturbance, though they may be somewhat more anxious immediately pre-operatively. The manner in which the information is imparted must match the patient's style of psychological defences, or there are negative effects.

79. Observing violence on television tends to have what effect(s) on children?

a) It produces more disturbing dreams
b) It has no effect on daytime behaviour
c) It stimulates temporary aggressive behaviour
d) It inhibits later aggressive behaviour
e) It increases enuresis

80. What are the characteristics of a Likert scale for the measurement of attitudes?

a) Each concept is judged on a series of bipolar semantic scales
b) A series of statements of attitude spaced equally along an attitude continuum are rated as 'agree' or 'disagree'
c) On a 5-point scale, one indicates the extent of one's agreement with a set of attitude statements
d) Responses to open-ended questions are coded by content analysis
e) One ticks all acceptable statements in a set of items arranged in order of difficulty of acceptance by the average subject

81. Which of these are true statements concerning concepts of schizophrenia?

a) Kraepelin originated the term 'schizophrenia'
b) Bleuler originated the term 'dementia praecox'
c) Schneider described first rank symptoms
d) Laing first described the 'double-bind' hypothesis of causation
e) All of the above

Answers overleaf

79. c)

Many studies have addressed this issue, in children from various backgrounds and of varying ages. It appears that a temporary stimulation of aggressive ideas and behaviour results.

80. c)

A Likert-type scale is where the ratings on each 5-point scale are added to give an over-all attitude score. It is less laborious to produce and use than the Thurstone technique (b) which requires a group of judges to agree on the sorting of the statements along the continuum; and the Guttman scalogram (e) which assumes a unidimensional concept and assumes that the items are cumulative (so agreement with any one implies agreement with all less extreme items on the scale). Osgood's semantic differential (a) presents a series of 7-point bipolar scales (e.g. dark–light, sweet–sour) answered with regard to an individual concept.

81. c)

a) and b). In 1896 Kraepelin defined dementia praecox and in 1911 Bleuler proposed the term 'schizophrenia', stressing the importance of the splitting of psychic functions.
c) Yes, though the concept of first rank symptoms confirming the diagnosis is now questioned.
d) No. Laing popularized this and other concepts, but did not originate it. Bateson and colleagues described this putatively causative mechanism. There is very little evidence that it does play a part in the causation of schizophrenia.
e) No.

CTP p. 298. *CPM* pp. 9, 35, 102. *GP* 339–40.

82. Which of these drugs does NOT produce an increased intracardiac conduction time?

a) Doxepin
b) Amitriptyline
c) Imipramine
d) Desipramine
e) Norpramine

83. The James-Lange theory of emotion proposes that the origin of the 'feelings' we experience as emotions is:

a) Changes in average arousal levels
b) Feedback from visceral organs
c) Simple conditioning
d) Activity within the thalamus
e) None of the above

84. Which of the following statements about the occurrence of schizophrenia is/are NOT true?

a) The occurrence in the general population is around 1%
b) The occurrence in parents of schizophrenics is around 5%
c) The occurrence in siblings of schizophrenics is around 25%
d) The occurrence in children of schizophrenics is around 10%
e) The concordance rate in monozygotic twins is around 30–40%

Answers overleaf

82. a)

Though it can disturb cardiac rhythm on overdosage, doxepin, unlike other tricyclic antidepressants, seems to have little effect on intracardiac conduction. In patients with intracardiac conduction defects, such as right bundle branch block, doxepin may be the preferable tricyclic.

Secunda S. (1980); Pinder R. M. *et al.* (1977).
CTP pp. 790, 793.

83. b)

The James–Lange theory is based on William James' idea that overt perception of the responses of visceral and somatic organs *is* the emotion: autonomic nervous system activity producing visceral and somatic responses which are perceived by the conscious mind as an emotion. Strong exception is taken to this point of view.

84. c)

(a) (b) (d) and (e) are true and are evidence supporting the view that genetic factors are important in the causation of schizophrenia; (c) is untrue, as the occurrence rate in siblings of schizophrenics is generally around 8%.

CTP pp. 302–4. *CPM* pp. 64, 162–3. *GP* pp. 341–2.

85. Physiological effects of placebo use can include all the following EXCEPT:
   a) relief of pain via endorphin release
   b) reduced rapid-eye-movement (REM) phase of sleep
   c) decreased gastric motility
   d) increased gastric acid secretion
   e) increased exercise-induced bronchospasm in asthmatics

86. Among patients with angina pectoris, what proportion can be expected to receive relief from a placebo?
   a) 1% to 2%
   b) 5% to 10%
   c) 20% to 40%
   d) 60% to 70%
   e) 80% to 90%

87. According to the 'gate control' theory of Melzack and Wall, pain perception can be diminished by:
   a) Acupuncture, especially in the cervical area
   b) Neocortical depolarization of afferent impulses to the hypothalamus
   c) Inhibitory impulses from the ventral nuclei to the thalamus
   d) Neocortical depolarization of afferent impulses to the spinal cord
   e) None of the above

Answers overleaf

85. e)

(a), (b) and (c) are all recognized physiological effects of placebo; (c) and (d)—gastric acid secretion and motility can be increased or decreased, depending on what the patient is told; (e) no, exercise-induced bronchospasm in asthmatics can be *decreased* in some 40% of patients.

Wolf S. (1973); Vogel A. V. *et al.* (1980).
GP pp. 558–9.

86. c)

Of patients with angina, 20% to 40% report relief from the use of a placebo; 30% to 40% of patients with pain after abdominal surgery, cough, or depression may respond similarly, around 50% of those complaining of anxiety; and 30% to 60% of those with headache respond well.

Wolf S. (1973); Vogel A. V. *et al.* (1980).

87. d)

The 'gate control' theory suggests that impulses from primary afferent neurons carrying pain messages to the spinal cord are blocked in the substantia gelatinosa by depolarizing impulses from the brain. Through this mechanism, cognitive and emotional factors can affect the intensity of pain perception.

GP pp. 154–5.

88. You are asked to evaluate the current suicide risk of a patient in casualty. He is a 23-year-old married biologist who has taken an overdose of 12 Aspirin. He says he wants to die, and has made a previous attempt two years ago. In the previous week he gave away his stereo and his tropical fish to friends. What is the most ominous factor in this history, indicating high lethality?

a) His age
b) His having given away his stereo
c) His occupation
d) His having used aspirin
e) His marital status

89. Symptoms of tardive dyskinesia

a) May occur spontaneously when no medication has been taken
b) Occur only after antipsychotic medications have been taken over long periods
c) Occur only in schizophrenic patients
d) Stop when the antipsychotic medication is discontinued
e) All of the above

90. A normal infant begins to show selective social smiling, responding to specific known faces at around the age of:

a) 1-2 weeks
b) 6-8 weeks
c) 18-20 weeks
d) 30-36 weeks
e) 40-48 weeks

Answers overleaf

88. b)

The giving away of valued personal possessions is a significant and ominous prognostic sign, like writing and executing one's own will. The lethality of the method chosen matters, and 12 aspirin are of relatively low lethality. Older men are more at risk; a male of this age is possibly of higher risk than a woman. Biologists are not an especially high risk group. Married men are less at risk than single or divorced/separated men. His previous attempt is relevant and somewhat adds to the risk rather than diminishes it.

Hatton C. L. *et al.* (1977).
CTP Chap. 27.1, pp. 704–10. *CPM* pp. 556–61. *GP* pp. 431, 434–6.

89. a)

b) and (c) False. Tardive dyskinesia may be idiopathic; it certainly is not limited to schizophrenics; it may be causally related, induced or worsened by other drugs, such as sympathomimetics, antihistamines, tricyclic antidepressants in high doses, possibly even diazepam.
d) False—the symptoms may not stop when medication is discontinued, and may even get worse.
e) False.
CTP pp. 785. *CPM* pp. 480–4. *GP* 531–3.

90. c)

A normal child usually smiles within the first or second week of life, but it is a natural non-specific response (blind infants also smile, at the same age). The first social smile, responding to the face or voice of someone else occurs sometime during the second month; and a selective social smile in response to a recognised familiar face or voice, at around 18–20 weeks.

CTP Chap. 30.1 pp. 834–41. *GP* pp. 463–70.

91. One of your patients asks for advice about giving sexual information to their child. Which of the following points of view would you support?

a) It is usually safe to give more, rather than less, information when in doubt
b) Always answer any question a child asks, fully and directly
c) The particular needs and vulnerabilities of each developmental stage are such that giving the wrong sexual information at the wrong stage may be dangerous
d) Giving information too early is over-stimulating and leads to experimentation
e) Sex play between children leads to adult sexual dysfunction

92. The intelligence quotient (IQ) expresses the relationship between the chronological age (CA) and the mental age (MA). Which formula best expresses this relationship?

a) $\frac{CA}{MA} - 100$

b) $\frac{MA}{100} \times CA$

c) $\frac{CA}{MA} \times 100$

d) $\frac{MA}{CA} - 100$

e) $\frac{MA}{CA} \times 100$

93. Which of the following statements about the incidences of depression is/are NOT true

a) The incidence in the general population is around 1%
b) The incidence in first degree relatives of depressed patients is around 10–15%
c) There is a concordance rate of 20% for dizygotic twins
d) There is a concordance rate of 70% for monozygotic twins
e) None of the above are true

Answers overleaf

91. a)

a) Yes. Experience and more formal studies agree quite consistently that a child will be likely to forget or not pay attention to anything he or she cannot understand, or in which he or she is not yet interested.

b) No. True, but not true enough. Children may not know enough to ask the questions they need to have answered, and may need help in articulating their concerns and curiosity. Also, their actual interest may be more limited than their question implies, and in the attempt to answer 'fully and directly', you may give far more information than the child wanted or can use. Finally, the question may be phrased cognitively, but may indicate a need for more emotional discussion than a factual answer.

c) No, though emotional characteristics and interests may vary developmentally, and cognitive growth will affect the child's way of conceptualizing complex phenomena; ignorance or misinformation causes far more emotional problems at any age than does knowledge. There is little evidence to suggest that any knowledge given with even minimal tact and sensitivity has ever caused a child any harm.

d) No, quite wrong. There is no evidence that accurate knowledge given sensibly causes any problems. The fantasies that may flourish in the absence of real information may be more harmful. There is no evidence that such knowledge leads to any more sexual activity than does fantasy, ignorance, secrecy and false beliefs, and it may help to protect them from being misled by others.

e) No. Exploration and play is normal and common, and there's no evidence of any link with later problems.

92. e)

In standard tests of the IQ, like the Stanford–Binet and Wechsler tests, scores allow one to calculate the mental age (an MA of 12 is a test performance equivalent to that of an average 12 year old). The relationship of MA divided by CA is expressed as a percentage. Thus the average IQ is 100 (when MA = CA).

CTP Chap. 10.5, pp. 205–8. *GP* p. 3.

93. e)

CTP p. 372.

94. Children with infantile autism usually show all of these features EXCEPT:

a) Panic when separated from mother
b) Limited eye contact
c) Stereotyped mannerisms
d) Obsessive need for sameness
e) Limited use of language for communication

95. Following an overdose of paracetamol (acetaminophen), early symptoms (within the first 24 hours) usually include all EXCEPT which of the following?

a) Nausea
b) Epigastric pain
c) Liver tenderness
d) Anorexia
e) Coma

96. Typical features of the Sturge–Weber syndrome include:

a) Polydactyly
b) Mental handicap
c) Venous angioma of pia
d) Phakomata
e) Hypertelorism

Answers overleaf

94. a)

This is almost incompatible with the diagnosis of autism, and sounds more typical of separation anxiety.
CTP pp. 870–2. *CPM* 625–30. (*GP* p. 339.)

95. e)

In the first 24 hours the patient may show anorexia, nausea and vomiting, epigastric pain and liver tenderness. Coma in the first day is hardly ever due to this drug, so other drugs or causes would be suspected. Jaundice may occur on the 3rd to 5th day after overdose.

96. b), c)

a) No, this is seen in the Laurence–Moon–Biedl syndrome.
b) Yes, also fits and possibly hemiplegia.
c) Yes, also naevi/portwine stains, especially on the face and neck.
d) No, these, with adenoma sebaceum, are features of tuberous sclerosis (epiloia).
e) No, though it may be associated with mental handicap, hypertelorism is an abnormality of the base of the skull, producing great breadth between the eyes.

CTP pp. 861–4. *CPM* p. 407. *GP* p. 443.

97. From the orthodox Freudian viewpoint, the super-ego contains the

a) pleasure principle
b) ego ideal
c) reality principle
d) conscience
e) the origins of the libido

98. In regard to postpartum or puerperal psychiatric problems:

a) Postpartum psychosis usually begins immediately after delivery
b) Postpartum 'blues' are very common
c) Cerebral thrombo–embolic lesions may be mistaken for postpartum psychosis
d) The prognosis for postpartum psychosis is different from that of similar affective or psychiatric illnesses arising at other times
e) The risk of recurrence in future pregnancies is 1 in 2

99. When prescribing antidepressant medication for suicidal patients, one should:

a) Monitor blood levels
b) Limit the amount of medication prescribed at one time
c) Use a more sedative antidepressant
d) Use a more activating antidepressant
e) Consider giving the medication to another family member for safe-keeping

Answers overleaf

97. b), d)

The Freudian super-ego contains the conscience (as a set of internalized moral views and prohibitions) and the ego ideal, an internalized set of positive values the ego tries to emulate.

CTP p. 136. *CPM* p. 20. *GP* p. 23.

98. b), c)

a) No, the mother is usually well for the first few days postpartum. The problem begins in the first month in 60% of cases, within 3 months in 80% of cases.

b) Yes, transient weepiness and poor concentration during the first week are common.

c) Yes, and it is important that the distinction be made early and clearly.

d) No, the treatment and prognosis are the same.

e) No, but there is a 1 in 5 risk of recurrence, more than 100 times the risk in the general population of postpartum women.

CTP Chap. 17.2, pp. 380–3. *CPM* p. 247.

99. b), e)

Blood level monitoring (a) or the nature of the antidepressant (c) and (d) will have little effect on suicide risk (except in so far as they relate to effective treatment of the depression). Limiting the amount of medication accessible to the patient at any one time (b) and enlisting the help of another family member (e) may help to reduce the risk.

Hatton C. L. *et al.* (1977).

100. Concerning noctural enuresis, which of these statements is/are UNTRUE?

a) There may be a strong family history
b) Diuretics are useful in its management
c) Urinary tract anomalies are uncommon
d) Conditioning may be useful in its management
e) It is rare over 10 years of age

101. According to Eccles and others, what are believed to be typical functions of the dominant cerebral hemisphere?

a) Musical
b) Sequential
c) Synthesis
d) Analogue
e) Verbal

102. Which of these are NOT lipid disorders associated with mental handicap:

a) Tay-Sachs disease
b) Hurler's syndrome
c) Gaucher's disease
d) Niemann-Pick disease
e) Laurence-Moon-Biedl syndrome

Answers overleaf

100. b), e)

a) Yes, there may be a strong family history of nocturnal enuresis.
b) Untrue, diuretics play no part in routine management.
c) Yes, imipramine, 25–50 mg at night, may be useful in older children.
d) Yes, conditioning using pad-and-bell type apparatus, may be useful.
e) Untrue. At 14 years of age, it still occurs in 1 in 35 children, even if it is far commoner in earlier years.

CTP Chap. 39.5 pp. 985–90. *GP* pp. 479–80.

101. b), e)

Dominant hemisphere functions are considered to include verbal, ideational, analytic, sequential, arithmatic and digital. Non-dominant hemisphere functions are regarded as including nonverbal and musical, pictorial and patterns, synthetic, holistic and non-linear, geometric and analogue.

102. b), e)

The lipid disorders concerned are inborn metabolic abnormalities, autosomal recessives, where an enzyme deficiency blocks a metabolic reaction, leading to an abnormal accumulation of lipids.
  a) Gaglioside lipids are affected.
  b) This is gargoylism, a connective tissue disorder. Though also an inborn metabolic anomaly associated with mental subnormality, this is not a lipid disorder.
  c) Cerebroside lipids are affected.
  d) Sphingomyelin lipids are affected.
  e) This is a neurological deficit also involving retardation, with polydactyly, hypogenitalism, obesity and retinal degeneration, but not a lipid disorder.

CTP Chap. 32, pp. 851–68, esp. 855-6. *CPM* Chap. 22 pp. 406-8. *GP* pp. 447-8.

103. **Which of the following statements about non-parametric statistical procedures are NOT true?**
   a) The population concerned must be normally distributed
   b) They are preferable to parametric techniques when the samples are smaller than 12
   c) Sample variates may not be discontinuous
   d) Variables must be measured with more than interval-level scales
   e) They test the hypothesis that the two (or more) population distributions are identical

104. **Diazepam may be contraindicated in patients with a history of:**
   a) Chronic anaemia
   b) Narrow angle glaucoma
   c) Psychomotor epilepsy
   d) Active duodenal ulcer
   e) Hypersensitivity to the drug

105. **Cardiovascular effects of phenothiazines do NOT include:**
   a) T-wave notching
   b) Q-T interval prolongation
   c) Bradyarrhythmias
   d) Postural hypertension
   e) Cardiomyopathy

Answers overleaf

103. a), d)

Non-parametric statistics are often used when it is not possible to meet the strict assumptions needed for proper application of parametric, classic, statistical procedures. They need make *no* assumptions about the population distribution shape, and in fact compare distributions rather than other parameters estimated from distributions. Interval-level measures are not needed, even nominal data can be used. The only assumption is that the variable must have no discontinuities.

Swinscow T. D. (1980); Robson C. (1973); Walizer M. H., Wienir P. L. (1978); Downie N. M., Starry, A. R. (1977).

104. b), e)

Obviously, hypersensitivity is a contraindication, and so is acute narrow-angle glaucoma (it can be used in patients with open angle glaucoma who are receiving appropriate therapy for it). It is not contraindicated in psychomotor epilepsy—it has been used in the management of epilepsy, though it has precipitated tonic status epilepticus in patients treated for petit mal status. It is not contraindicated in active duodenal ulcer.

105. c), d)

T-wave notching (a) and QT-interval prolongation (b) are the chief electrocardiographic effects, more common and more marked with the aliphatic and piperidyl than with the piperazine phenothiazines. These changes occur in nearly 100% of patients on some of these drugs at normal therapeutic doses, and may be reversed by potassium ingestion; (c) and (d) are wrong—tachyarrhythmias (which may respond to propranolol) and postural hypotension occur; (e) significant cardiomyopathy can occur, though not common. Myocardial changes appear similar to those seen in alcoholic cardiomyopathy.

106. In schizophrenia, which of these factors is considered to be associated with an unfavorable prognosis?

a) Slow onset of the disorder
b) Presence of depressive features
c) Relatively high intelligence
d) An external precipitating event
e) Inappropriate or flat affect

107. Among people regularly taking large doses of amphetamines, which of the following is/are true:

a) Hallucinations are common
b) A condition resembling depression is common
c) A psychosis resembling catatonic schizophrenia occurs
d) A psychosis resembling paranoid schizophrenia is quite common
e) Repeated episodes of *déjà vécu* occur

108. According to crisis theory, crisis intervention may be effective because:

a) Profound intrapsychic dynamic change is possible during crisis
b) The patient feels the need for help more urgently
c) The adaptive capacities of the individual can be enhanced to help him deal better with similar stresses in the future
d) The second six months of treatment can build on changes achieved in the first six months
e) All of the above

Answers overleaf

106. a), e)

Slow, rather than acute onset of the condition, and inappropriate or flat affect, are regarded as unfavourable prognostic signs. Other features suggesting a better prognosis include preservation of normal affect or depressive features, relatively high intelligence, evidence of a precipitating event, age under 30 at onset, and a history of good emotional adjustment prior to the onset.

CTP pp. 332. *CPM* p. 176. *GP* pp. 376-7.

107. a), d)

Especially at doses over 50 mg per day, hallucinations are common and a psychosis resembling paranoid schizophrenia, with persecutory delusions in a clear sensorium, is quite common. Usually the psychosis subsides gradually after the drug use stops.

CTP pp. 515-516. *CPM* pp. 568-569. *GP* 229-30.

108. b), c)

a) No, major dynamic change is neither expected nor sought after; the main emphasis is on maintaining and strengthening the status quo prior to the crisis.
b) and c) are right, as these are considered to be advantages of this approach.
d) No, it is very uncommon for such therapy to last longer than two months. Longer interventions do not constitute crisis intervention.
e) is therefore not correct.

CTP Chap. 28.7, pp. 766-70. *CPM* Chap. 27, pp. 542-51. *GP* p. 593.

109. Pseudodementia is:

a) Characterized by memory loss
b) Caused by stroke
c) Characterized by an abnormal EEG
d) Rarely reversible
e) Often improves when treated with antidepressants or ECT

110. Traits related to the anal stage within the Freudian developmental model include all of these EXCEPT:

a) Punctuality
b) Curiosity
c) Frugality
d) Stubborness
e) Orderliness

111. At one year of age, the average child can:

a) Stand alone briefly
b) Dress and undress himself
c) Walk with one hand held
d) Have complete sphincter control
e) None of above

Answers overleaf

109. a), e)

Pseudodementia, or the dementia syndrome, of depression can be distinguished from Alzheimer's disease or other causes by an onset with depressive features, an acute course, often a previous or family history of manic-depressive disorder, an absence of localizing neurological findings, and usually a normal EEG. The cognitive disorder can be as severe as that found in Alzheimer's disease, and patients run all the risks of any dementia unless proper antidepressive treatment is initiated.

CTP p. 395. *CPM* p. 283. *GP* pp. 94–5, 326.

110. b)

Curiosity is not a trait associated with the anal stage of development, the successful resolution of which forms the basis of personal autonomy and initiative. Fixation at this stage produces more parsimony, willfulness, orderliness, obstinacy and stubbornness.

CTP Chap. 6, pp. 123–8. *GP* p. 22.

111. a), c)

b) Wrong—such a child can cooperate in dressing, but cannot do it alone.

d) and e) Incorrect. A child of five can dress independently and has complete sphincter control, but not a child of one.

CTP Chap. 30.1, pp. 834–41. *GP* pp. 463–70.

112. Factors commonly associated with poor treatment compliance include:

a) Complex treatment regimes
b) Involvement of other health professionals in treatment
c) Anxiety during the consultation
d) Clear definition of treatment goals
e) Severe warning of the consequences of treatment failure

113. Bilateral temporal lobe lesions in monkeys produces the Kluver–Bucy syndrome, characterized by:

a) Hyposexuality
b) Hyperphagia
c) Docility
d) Rage attacks
e) Hypophagia

114. Of drugs metabolized on first-pass, which of the following statements is/are true?

a) Nitroglycerin is an example
b) They are not effective clinically
c) They are almost completely metabolized in the liver on their first circulation through it
d) Methaqualone is an example
e) They may be metabolized into more active metabolites

Answers overleaf

112. a), c)

a) Yes, the more complex the treatment regime, and the more tablets that need to be taken, the poorer the compliance.
b) No, involvement of other health professionals in treatment tends to improve compliance, if it has any effect.
c) Yes, anxiety during the consultation decreases understanding and remembering.
d) No, clear definition of goals helps.
e) No, severe warnings do not help, they increase anxiety and decrease compliance.

Blackwell B. (1979); Haynes R. B. *et al.* (1979).

113. b), c)

Bilateral temporal lobectomy (involving amydala, hippocampus, parahippocampal gyrus, and temporal cortex) produces the Kluver–Bucy syndrome in monkeys. Typical features include hypersexuality, hyperphagia, docility, visual agnosia, and compulsive oral activity. Similar though modified symptoms, plus serious memory loss, can occur in humans with bilateral temporal lobe lesions.

CTP p. 34. *CPM* p. 36.

114. a), c), e)

a) Yes—to get effective serum levels, it must be taken sublingually. Taken orally, even doses 10 times larger do not give comparable steady levels.
b) No, they can be effective either when taken by a different route, as with nitroglycerin, or, as with acetylsalicylic acid and propranolol, because the metabolites are themselves active agents.
c) Yes, this is the definition of a first-pass drug.
d) No, it shows second-order kinetics.
e) Yes, such as acetylsalicylic acid and propranolol, as described above.

Melman K. L., Morrelli H. F. (1978); Bochner F. *et al.* (1978).

115. Which of these comments on school phobia are NOT true?

a) It may present with abdominal pain
b) It occurs more often in girls than boys
c) It often occurs in children who also show truancy
d) The mother is often over-protective
e) It is more often related to separation anxiety than to fear of school

116. In managing mild symptoms of phencyclidine (PCP) intoxication, it would be INAPPROPRIATE to:

a) Administer a barbiturate sedative
b) Maintain adequate urinary flow
c) Maintain minimal sensory stimuli in the patient's environment
d) Acidify urine with ascorbic acid, keeping urine pH below 5 for a week
e) Administer chlorpromazine

117. When using tricyclic antidepressants (TCAs) in cardiac patients, which of these comments are NOT true:

a) The dosage of quinidine or procainamide must be lowered when TCAs are prescribed
b) In right or left bundle branch block and depression, Doxepin may be the preferable TCA
c) An initial, base-line ECG should be taken
d) TCAs block the antihypertensive effect of guanethidine and clonidine
e) TCAs have no direct myocardial depressant effect.

Answers overleaf

115. b), c)

a) Yes, it may present with abdominal pain or nausea.
b) Untrue, school phobia is more common in boys than in girls.
c) Untrue, school phobia is quite distinct from truancy. It often occurs in children who are doing well at school.
d) Yes, over-protective mothers who may themselves be prone to depression, are quite commonly a part of the clinical picture.
e) Yes. Involvement of the family in therapy may be important.

CTP p. 723. *CPM* pp. 611–2.

116. a), e)

Acidifying urine and maintaining urinary flow will aid excretion of PCP; minimizing sensory stimulation may help to reduce agitation. One should also monitor vital signs and fluid balance; repeating electrolytes, blood pH and blood gases. Barbiturate and chlorpromazine are not advised in the management of PCP intoxication.

CTP pp. 406, 720. *CPM* p. 219. *GP* p. 494.

117. e)

a) Yes, they have quinidine-like effects in their own right, in delay of cardiac conduction—they have even been suggested as potentially useful in depressed patients with premature depolarizations.
b) Yes, as TCAs may cause delay in intracardiac conduction, as said above.
c) Yes, to be able to evaluate possible later changes in ECG.
d) Yes.
e) No. TCAs certainly do have a direct myocardial depressant effect, and may exacerbate heart failure.

118. Which of these statements about mental retardation are UNTRUE? Someone with:

a) An IQ of 95 would be classified as mildly retarded
b) An IQ of 45 would be classified as moderately retarded
c) An IQ of 25 would be classified as severely retarded
d) An IQ of 15 would be classified as profoundly retarded
e) An IQ of 105 would be regarded as normal

119. A serum bromide level would be an appropriate investigation in a patient who complains of unexplained:

a) Auditory hallucinations
b) Delusions
c) Epileptic fits
d) Bilateral numbness in the hands
e) Foot drop

120. You may be asked to evaluate a patient's ability to make out a valid will, which is referred to as:

a) Testamentary capacity
b) Responsibility
c) Competency
d) Functional commitment
e) Sanity

Answers overleaf

118. b), c), d), e)

a) No. Mild retardation means an IQ under 75; an IQ of 95 is normal and common. For every case of severe retardation there are estimated to be four moderate, and fifteen mild cases.

CTP Chap. 32, pp. 851–68. *CPM* Chap. 22, pp. 400–19. *GP* pp. 439–61.

119. a), b)

Bromism may present with various symptoms, including auditory and visual hallucinations, delusions, marked emotional lability, lethargy or hypomania, headaches, depression, acne-like skin rash on the face and at the hair margins, and bad breath.

CTP p. 405. *CPM* pp. 295–6, 565–6. *GP* pp. 143–4.

120. a)

The specific capacity to make a valid will is called testamentary capacity. Competency is a general term for a person's ability to make decisions or perform specific functions competently. It is assessed in law in relation to the particular function (such as capacity to sign a contract, to embark on marriage or divorce). Responsibility is a term sometimes used in relation to criminal conduct. Sanity is a term used in law, in rhetorical arguments, and by Thomas Szasz. It is not a psychiatric term at all. As Groucho Marx said: 'There ain't no sanity clause'.

CTP Chap. 43 pp. 1023–34. *CPM* Chap. 34 pp. 665–97. *GP* pp. 632–3.

121. The major form of toxicity following acute overdose of paracetomol (acetaminophen USA) is:
   a) Early status epilepticus
   b) Hepatotoxicity
   c) Nephropathy
   d) Hypothermia
   e) Tinnitus

122. The principles of operant conditioning suggest that a behaviour will be maintained, at a constant or increasing frequency, only if it is:
   a) Unconditioned
   b) Adaptive
   c) Periodically reinforced
   d) Not punished
   e) Stimulus-specific

123. All of the following are ego defense mechanisms according to psychoanalytic theory, EXCEPT:
   a) Cathexis
   b) Projection
   c) Repression
   d) Reaction-formation
   e) Undoing

Answers overleaf

81

121. b)

Hepatotoxicity is the major risk. Jaundice may occur 3 to 5 days after the overdose, and hepatic encephalopathy may occur. Disseminated intravascular coagulopathy may ensue, and coma, gastro-intestinal bleeding and cardiac arrhythmias may attend death from the overdose.

Ameer B. Greenblatt D. J. (1977).

122. c)

Periodic reinforcement is regarded as necessary.

Wolpe J. (1973).
CTP Chap. 28.2 pp. 743-7. *GP* pp. 4-5.

123. a)

Cathexis refers to the investment of libido in an object. Among the principle ego defenses recognized in the work of Sigmund and Anna Freud are introjection, regression, repression, reaction-formation, isolation, projection, reversal, and undoing.

Freud A. (1946).
CTP pp. 137-8. *CPM* pp. 20-1. *GP* pp. 26-9, 352-3.

124. A probable contradiction to the use of propranolol in the management of anxiety in a patient would be the patient's history of:

a) Asthma
b) Allergy
c) Hypertension
d) Cardiac arrythmias
e) Constipation

125. Which aspect of a person's results will probably increase during psychological testing due to fatigue, boredom, distraction and low motivation?

a) Validity
b) Type I error
c) Type II error
d) Random error
e) Reliability

126. The hormone whose role in relation to aggression is best established is:

a) Oestrogen
b) Testosterone
c) Aldosterone
d) Progesterone
e) Thyroxine

Answers overleaf

124. a)

Propranolol, a β-adrenergic receptor blocker, may be used in the management of hypertension and arrhythmias, so these are not contraindications. But asthma can be a predictable and possibly serious side-effect in some individuals, and can constitute a contraindication to its use. It can produce a slowing of the pulse, reduction of palpitations, reduction of amplitude of muscle tremor, etc. Allergy and constipation are not contraindications.

CTP p. 833. *CPM* pp. 393–4, 492–3.

125. d)

Random error increases under these circumstances.

126. b)

In many animal species, the male shows more aggressive behaviour than the female, and castration generally reduces aggression. If testosterone is experimentally administered post-puberty to previously castrated male rats, they may return to normal levels of aggressiveness. Young female mice reared on androgens develop otherwise uncharacteristic aggressive behaviour.

CTP Chap. 3.4, pp. 66–71.

127. In the Capgras syndrome, the patient evinces a delusional belief that:
   a) He is changing into a member of the opposite sex
   b) He has a sexual relationship with a very famous person
   c) Significant people in his life have been secretly replaced by imposters
   d) People are plotting to harm him
   e) He is pregnant

128. Common side-effects of phenytoin include:
   a) Gum hyperplasia
   b) Acne
   c) Hypomagnesaemia
   d) Tolerance
   e) Polycythaemia

129. Components of the Wechsler Adult Intelligence Scale (WAIS) include all of these EXCEPT:
   a) Picture Completion
   b) Block Design
   c) Digit Span
   d) Thematic Apperception
   e) Vocabulary

Answers overleaf

127. c)

b) This is De Clerambault's syndrome.
Enoch M. D., Trethowan W.H. (1979)
CTP pp. 238, 658. *CPM p. 422.*

128. a), b)

Among the recognized side-effects of phenytoin are vestibular/cerebellar disturbances, diffuse encephalopathy, gum hyperplasia, acne, excess hair growth, and a megaloblastic anaemia (reversable with folic acid).
CTP p. 406. *CPM* p. 249. *GP* pp. 120-1.

129. d)

a) Yes, this involves noticing missing items in pictures.
b) Yes, this involves reproducing specified designs, using coloured blocks.
c) Yes, this involves remembering increasing sequences of numbers.
d) No, the Thematic Apperception Test (TAT) is a projective personality test in which you are asked to report what you perceive in ambiguous pictures.
e) Yes, it involves defining words of increasing difficulty. The WAIS includes 11 sub-tests, 6 verbal (including (c) and (e), and 5 performance (including (a) and (b)).
CTP pp. 206, 208, 217. *GP* p. 12.

130. When a physician's feelings about a patient are aroused, based on resemblances to significant people in the physician's life, it is called:
a) Transference
b) Projection
c) Identification
d) Displacement
e) Countertransference

131. Which of these is a quadricyclic antidepressant compound?
a) Trazodone
b) Nomifensive
c) Buproprione
d) Mianserin
e) Maprotiline

132. Carl Jung described the concept of:
a) Organ inferiority
b) The collective unconscious
c) Ego defense mechanisms
d) Cyclothymia
e) The distinction between dementia praecox and manic depressive psychosis

Answers overleaf

130. e)

A doctor's feelings for a patient may not always be based on the reality of who the patient is and what the patient is doing, but may be related to the patient's resemblances to an important person in the doctor's own earlier life, and this is called countertransference. The feelings may be positive or negative. There are of course also good objective reasons for liking or disliking some patients. But if one feels particularly antagonistic towards some types of patients, one should seek to understand what is so bothersome and how it may relate to one's own unresolved conflicts.

CTP pp. 177-8, 730. *GP* p. 566.

131. d)

Mianserin is a quadricyclic. Nomifensine has significant dopaminergic effect; Trazodone acts predominantly in the serotonergic system.

132. b)

Jung described the collective unconscious. Alfred Adler described the concept of organ inferiority. Ego defense mechanisms were described by Sigmund and Anna Freud. The term 'cyclothymic personality' or 'cyclothymia' was introduced by Kahlbaum. The distinction between dementia praecox and manic depressive psychosis was made by Kraepelin.

CTP Chaps. 1.1, 8.3. *CPM* pp. 12-13, 22-4. *GP* pp. 30-1.

133. Neuroleptic drugs are thought to exert their antischizophrenic actions by blocking receptors for:
   a) Noradrenaline (norepinephrine)
   b) Serotonin
   c) Dopamine
   d) Enkephalin
   e) Acetylcholine

134. Human–growth–hormone secretion can be affected by numerous factors. Which of the following statements are correct?
   a) Basal HGH levels are consistently below normal in depressed patients
   b) Insulin-induced hypoglycaemia is a widely used procedure for inhibiting HGH release
   c) HGH response to hypoglycaemia is significantly diminished in emotionally normal postmenopausal women
   d) All of the above
   e) None of the above

135. On testing the pupillary light reflexes, you find the right eye reacts directly but not consensually. The left eye reacts consensually but not directly. There are no palsies of extraocular muscles. You suspect a lesion—where?
   a) Right optic tract
   b) Left optic tract
   c) Right optic nerve
   d) Left Edinger–Westphal nucleus
   e) Left optic nerve

Answers overleaf

133. c)

Dopamine—receptor blockade is not thought to be important in the antischizophrenic action of neuroleptic drugs.

CTP p. 41. *CPM* p. 40. *GP*.
Snyder S. H. (1979).

134. a)

(b) False—insulin-induced hypoglycaemia is used to stimulate HGH release; (c) False—HGH response to hypoglycaemia is significantly diminished in postmenopausal women suffering from a primary unipolar depressive illness, as compared with normal postmenopausal women; (d) and (e) are false.

Carrol B. J., Mendels J. (1976).
CPM pp. 138–9.

135. e)

The lesion is likely to be in the left optic nerve.

Walton J. N. (1977).

136. Anaesthesia and muscle relaxants are used in ECT, DECREASING the risk of:

a) Memory loss
b) Aspiration pneumonia
c) Cardiac arrhythmias
d) Compression fractures
e) Hypertension

137. According to Freudian theory, children pass through each of the following stages of psychosexual development EXCEPT for one. Which one?

a) Anal
b) Phallic
c) Autoerotic
d) Oral
e) Genital

138. After his baby sister was born, 6-year-old Jeff began sucking his thumb and wetting his bed, behaviours he had 'grown out of' long before. This is an instance of:

a) Reaction formation
b) Regression
c) Acting out
d) Jealousy
e) Compensation

Answers overleaf

136. d)

A primary advantage of the use of anaesthesia and muscle relaxants in ECT is the reduced incidence of compression fractures, as well as reducing the unpleasantness of the experience.

CTP Chap. 29.5 pp. 818–22. *CPM* Chap. 26, pp. 531–6. *GP* pp. 607–16.

137. c)

'Autoerotic' is not one of the Freudian stages. The psychosexual stages of development are characterized by the most significant erogenous zone during that period and include (a), (b), (d) and (e).

CTP pp. 124–8. (*GP* p. 22.)

138. b)

This is an example of regression, returning to more infantile behaviours.

CTP pp. 137. *GP* p. 22.

139. **Which anticonvulsant drug should NOT be used in combination with primidone?**
   a) Carbamazepine
   b) Diazepam
   c) Phenytoin
   d) Phenobarbital
   e) All of the above

140. **Each of these hormones are considered to have significant effects in influencing sexual behaviour, with which exception(s)?**
   a) Oxytocin
   b) Testosterone
   c) Androsterone
   d) Oestradiol
   e) Luteinizing hormone releasing factor (LHRF)

141. **A man of 49 is recovering from an acute myocardial infarction. On his 2nd day in the coronary care unit you are asked for a consultation. He appears confused and agitated, complains that people are talking to him and about him all night. Clinical examination, and investigations (including arterial blood gas and electrolyte estimates), seem to rule out organic causes for this state. Effective management would be:**
   a) Oral amitriptyline 25 mg t.d.s increasing to 150 mg per day
   b) Ignore the complaints, which will subside within a few days
   c) Intravenous haloperidol 2 mg, repeated as needed
   d) Intravenous diazepam 10 mg, repeated as needed
   e) Intramuscular chlorpromazine 50 mg, repeated as necessary

Answers overleaf

139. d)

Primidone could be combined with phenytoin, for example. But as it is partially metabolized to phenobarbital, there is an increased risk of cumulation of this drug, even to toxic levels, especially in children. Toxic effects might include dizziness, drowsiness, nausea or vomiting, vertigo, diplopia; more rarely a megaloblastic anaemia or lupus erythematosis.

CTP p. 407. *CPM* p. 373. *GP* pp. 119-25.

140. a)

Oxytocin is an apparently behaviourally inactive peptide hormone, serving mainly to influence uterine contractions in parturition, and milk ejection in lactation. The others, gonadal steroids, do influence sexual behaviour and have been shown in a variety of mammalian species to be needed for the development of appropriate reproductive and parenting behaviour.

CPM pp. 47-8.

141. c)

This is the best advice. Optimal management, with a lower incidence of troublesome side-effects, would probably be achieved with haloperidol. Dystonic, extra-pyramidal reactions are possible. One should not ignore his complaints, as the confusion and agitation can seriously complicate his condition. Diazepam and chlorpromazine could be used, though diazepam would be less effective in clearing the confusional state rather than simply calming the agitation, and chlorpromazine could be more sedating than one would wish. There is no indication for the use of amitriptyline and its possible effect on cardiac conduction would give rise to concern.

142. Which of these statements is/are NOT true of the double-bind situation?

a) Two conflicting messages are given simultaneously
b) One message is often verbal, while the other is nonverbal
c) It has been clearly shown to be a cause of schizophrenia
d) It requires a response, when no 'correct' response is possible
e) Meta-communication and comments on the situation itself are not allowed

143. Which of the following side-effects of antipsychotic medications occur LESS frequently in the elderly?

a) Anticholinergic effects
b) Tardive dyskinesia
c) Hypotensive reactions
d) Dystonic reactions
e) None of the above

144. *Folie du doute* is typical of:

a) Paranoia
b) Obsessive–compulsive neurosis
c) Hysteria
d) Schizophrenia
e) Organic brain syndromes

Answers overleaf

142. c)

This is the correct response, for it is wrong. Double-bind situations may be significantly stressful, though far more ubiquitous and less specifically schizophrenogenic than originally described by Bateson, Jackson, Haley and Weakland.

GP p. 352.

143. d)

Dystonic reactions occur rather less frequently in the elderly.

Birren J., Sloan R. R. (1980); Busse E., Blazer D. (1980).

144. b)

Folie du doute is typical of obsessive–compulsive neurosis, and characterized by persistent doubting, indecisiveness and vacillation.

CTP p. 444. *GP* p. 309.

145. Barbiturates:

a) Decrease plasma levels of tricyclics
b) Increase plasma levels of phenothiazines
c) Tend to produce liver enzyme induction
d) Should be administered along with phenothiazines to reduce side-effects
e) All of the above

146. In follow-up studies reported by Masters and Johnson, and other sex therapists, which of the following varieties of sexual dysfunction has the lowest rate of cure?

a) Vaginismus
b) Premature ejaculation
c) Female orgasmic dysfunction
d) Primary impotence
e) Secondary impotence

147. Which of these statements about the Id are NOT consistent with psychoanalytic theory?

a) It is an area of mental life repressed by the Ego
b) It typifies secondary process thinking
c) It operates according to the pleasure principle
d) It is a primitive and unconscious mental structure
e) It is capable of hallucinatory wish-fulfillment

Answers overleaf

145. a), c)

Plasma levels of tricylics *and* phenothiazines can be decreased, both due to enzyme induction (c); (d) would not reduce side-effects usefully, probably only adding barbiturate risks and side-effects, and reducing efficacy of treatment.

146. d)

Masters and Johnson, and others, have reported in a 5-year follow-up study, rates of cure of almost 100% for vaginismus and premature ejaculation, and cure rates of 70% to 80% for female orgasmic dysfunction and secondary impotence. Treatment of primary impotence showed only a 60% rate of success. Recent failures to replicate these findings have cast some doubt on this earlier work.

Masters W. H., Johnson V. E. (1970).
CTP p. 570.

147. b)

The functions of the Id typify primary process thinking, characterized by illogical and atemporal operations, condensation and displacement, the pleasure-principle and wish-fulfilment.

CTP p. 132–3. *CPM* p. 20. *GP* pp. 22–3.

148. At what blood alcohol level would one expect a person to be in state of arousable stupor?

a) 25–75 mg %
b) 100–150 mg %
c) 150–250 mg %
d) 250–350 mg %
e) 350–500 mg %

149. Which of these structures are NOT included in the limbic system?

a) Corpus callosum
b) Hippocampus
c) Amygdala
d) Cingulate gyrus
e) Septal nuclei

150. Memory disturbance by convulsive therapy is least when the convulsion is induced by:

a) Indoklon
b) Bilateral ECT
c) Unilateral ECT over the dominant hemisphere
d) Unilateral ECT over the non-dominant hemisphere
e) Bilateral ECT with hyperoxygenation

Answers overleaf

148. d)

a) 25–75 mg %—No, relaxation and decreased inhibitions would be the likely effect.
b) 100–150 mg %—No, some limb ataxia and dysarthria may occur.
c) 150–250 mg %—No, some truncal ataxia and sleepiness can occur.
d) 250–350 mg %—Yes, arousable stupor would be typical.
e) 350–500 mg %—No, coma would be likely, and at levels of 500 to 800 mg % death can occur.

In some individuals highly tolerant to alcohol, comparable effects may occur at levels 100 to 200 mg % higher.

CTP Chap. 21.3. *CPM* Chap. 9 pp. 186–212.

149. a)

The limbic system, first described by Papez, is usually considered to include the cingulate and parahippocampal gyri, the hippocampus, amydala, and septal nuclei. It does not include the corpus callosum, though that structure runs through it, connecting the hemispheres.

CPM Chap. 3, pp. 35–7, *GP* p. 513.

150. d)

Unilateral ECT over the non-dominant hemisphere generally produces least memory disturbance. The inhalant convulsive Indoklon causes about as much confusion as bilateral ECT.

CTP Chap. 29.5, pp. 818–22. *CPM* Chap. 26, pp. 531–6. *GP* p. 615.

151. In the theories of Melanie Klein, the principle task in child development after the first year relates to:

 a) The depressive position
 b) The paranoid–schizoid position
 c) Projective identification
 d) Introjective identification
 e) Counter cathexis

152. Which of the following clinical features would be most significant in distinguishing between schizophrenia and an acute organic brain syndrome/delirium

 a) Difficulty in sustaining attention
 b) Fluctuation of level of consciousness
 c) Visual hallucinations
 d) Inappropriate affect
 e) Auditory hallucinations

153. A 15-year-old boy is recovering from severe brain trauma following a motor vehicle accident. He has poor short and intermediate-term memory and limited coordination The nurses complain that he has been masturbating in the presence of other patients and hospital staff. As a consultant, what responses would you recommend during the first week

 a) Physical restraints, such as wrist cuffs or straps
 b) A behaviour modification programme, rewarding appropriate behaviour and ignoring inappropriate behaviours
 c) Providing privacy for masturbation
 d) Sedation with chlorpromazine or diazepam
 e) Explaining to the patient why such behaviour is inappropriate

Answers overleaf

151. a)

The depressive position is the principle task. The paranoid–schizoid position occurs in the first six months, with splitting and projective identification as characteristic defenses. Anxiety for the child centres on the survival of his good objects, whereas earlier it had centred on his own survival.

CTP Chap. 8.5, pp. 162–3.

152. b)

Patients with acute organic brain syndrome (delirium) may have many symptoms resembling those of schizophrenia, including perceptual distortions, delusions, illusions, fluctuating attention, inappropriate affect, visual and auditory hallucinations. Generally, though, a fluctuating level of consciousness differentiates the two—in acute brain syndrome, which is due to altered brain metabolism, the level of consciousness fluctuates. Symptoms are often worse at night, partly due to loss of sensory clues which help to maintain orientation.

CTP Chap. 18, pp. 388–95. *CPM* Chap. 12 pp. 266–73.

153. c)

a) No, restraints will not stop inappropriate behaviours though they may alter or limit them; and may produce further behaviour problems. Restraints should be reserved for the protection of unalterably irrational self-injuring patients.
b) Probably not. Although this may occasionally be useful in such cases, the patient must have the capacity for immediate and intermediate recall in order to appreciate positive reinforcement as a reward for the behaviour that preceded it. Such an approach would probably not work in this case.
c) Yes, providing a private room allowing privacy for masturbation while rehabilitation and reassessment proceeds, would be wise. Anti-androgen medication could also be helpful.
d) No, the dosage needed to inhibit masturbation would probably produce major sedation interfering with many other mental and physical functions.
e) No, this is hardly likely to improve the situation.

154. In some patients with depression, which of the following have been demonstrated?
a) Maximal suppression of plasma cortisol levels following the administration of dexamethasone
b) A decreased number of cortisol-secretory episodes
c) No night-time cortisol secretion
d) Increased plasma cortisol concentration
e) None of the above

155. Pheromones are:
a) Chromosomes influencing emotional responses
b) Pituitary prohormones
c) Odorant molecules with behavioural effects
d) Enkephalin precursors
e) None of the above

156. In studies of aging, the theory of disengagement has been proposed, which refers to:
a) The ill-effects of retirement
b) The decrease in marital satisfaction with age
c) The decreasing capacity of older persons to care for themselves
d) The withdrawal of emotional commitment to the outside world by older persons
e) The tendency of children to increasingly neglect older parents

Answers overleaf

154. d)

a) Untrue. There are abnormalities of response to the dexamethasone suppression test. The typical response, first called 'non-suppression', is in fact an 'early escape' from suppression—but a lesser, graded response rather than maximal suppression.

b) Untrue. There are an increased number of secretary episodes, and an increase in the amount of time per day during which cortisol secretion occurs.

c) Untrue. There is active night-time cortisol secretion, whether the patient is asleep or awake.

d) Correct—as a result of the effects described in (b) and (c), there is an increase in plasma cortisol concentration, (e) is thus incorrect.

CTP p. 794. CPM p. 138.

155. c)

The term, originally used for chemicals used by social insects for communication functions, is now used for any specific chemical one organism produced that influences the responses of another organism of that species. Pheromones have been shown to influence human behaviour; and include responses to sweat and other body odours, bathing, deodorants and perfumes.

156. d)

The theory of disengagement, advanced by Cumming and Henry and others, refers to the withdrawal of interest in and concern with the environment that may occur in older people, their world shrinking as they become more concerned about their own immediate needs and less in the affairs of society.

157. In Abraham Maslow's use of the term 'self-actualization' to describe the adult capacity to realize one's full potential, which of the following is NOT a characteristic of the self-actualized person?

a) Creativity
b) Many close friends
c) Spontaneity
d) Autonomy
e) Unaffectedness

158. The necessary element for the antidepressant effects of electroconvulsive therapy (ECT) is believed to be:

a) The patient's expectation of therapeutic benefit
b) The patient's guilt and wish for punishment
c) The production of convulsions
d) The magnitude of the electronic impulse
e) The loss of memory following a shock

159. Which of the following are NOT varieties of personality disorder?

a) Cyclothymic
b) Anankastic
c) Borderline
d) Schizoid
e) Palimpsest

Answers overleaf

157. b)

In studying the lives of notable individuals he regarded as 'self-actualized', Maslow delineated all of the characteristics described here—except that these people were very selective in their friendships and tended to have only a few close friends.

CTP p. 167.

158. c)

Antidepressant efficacy of ECT depends on the occurrence of a convulsion (even if modified by succinylcholine and anaesthetic). Subconvulsive electrical stimulation can produce loss of consciousness and memory loss, but does not affect depression. The patient's expectations or guilt do not affect outcome significantly. Convulsions, whether electrically or chemically induced, have a therapeutic effect on depression.

CTP Chap. 29.5, pp. 818-2. *CPM* Chap. 26, pp. 531-7. *GP* pp. 607-16.

159. e)

a) Yes.

b) Yes, this is an old-fashioned alternative term for the obsessional personality.

c) Yes, this is an important variety of personality disorder, unjustifiably neglected in British psychiatry.

d) Yes.

e) No, this is a silly and illiterate term used by some in the field of alcoholism to describe a variety of memory disorder and false memory occurring in alcoholism. The term should not be used.

CTP Chap. 20, pp. 474-95. *CPM* Chap. 21, pp. 376-88. *GP* pp. 262-74.

160. In the cardiac or hypertensive patient, which of these statements are generally true?

a) Antihypertensive medication may have detrimental effects on sexual function
b) Introgenetic disturbance of sexual function is common in such cases
c) Masturbation is safer than intercourse
d) Sex after a myocardial infarction should be avoided
e) Sudden death during intercourse is relatively common

161. Lidz introduced the terms 'schismatic' and 'skewed' to describe:

a) Pathological interaction patterns in certain families
b) Superego deficits typical of sociopathy
c) Developmental anomalies in retarded children
d) Varieties of parataxis
e) Effects of countertransference in the therapy session

162. What is the most common finding on EEG one week after completion of a standard course of ECT treatments?

a) A normal record
b) Epileptiform activity
c) Focal slowing
d) Generalized slowing
e) Wave-and-spike

Answers overleaf

160. a), b)

a) Yes, the arousal phase of the sexual response is under mainly parasympathetic control, and the orgasmic phase under mainly sympathetic control, so drugs with autonomic actions are clearly able to interfere with function. Guanethidine, for example, as an adrenergic blocker, can inhibit ejaculation in men and orgasm in women.

b) Yes, vague or uncertain advice, lack of clear positive support for continuing sexual activity, and ominous comments like: 'take it easy with sex', all cause excess anxiety or fearful cessation of sexual activity.

c) No, there may not be much difference, but the physiological changes during sex are usually greater during masturbation than during intercourse.

d) No, once a patient can walk up two flights of stairs without major decompensation or angina, sex can safely be resumed. It can be useful exercise, and less energetic positions may be preferred. Avoiding sex may be more stressful and harmful

e) No, this is rare. There is some evidence that this rare event is commoner during extramarital intercourse.

161. a)

In the skewed family, family dynamics are distorted in the direction of one disturbed parent whose illness is often not openly acknowledged. In schismatic families the child is caught between two warring camps.

CPM p. 64.

162. d)

Electrophysiologically, a typical course of ECT results in the development of generalized slowing in the electroencephalogram (EEG). It does not produce focal or typically epileptiform activity.

CTP Chap. 29.5, pp. 818–22. *CPM* Chap. 26, pp. 531–7.

163. When a patient repeatedly turns the topic away from what appear to be highly relevant issues, switching to irrelevant topics during a therapy session, this may be an example of:

a) Projection
b) Resistance
c) Suppression
d) Repression
e) Denial

164. A typical presentation of tardive dyskinesia in an elderly patient:

a) Affects the jaws and lips but not the tongue
b) Is more obvious in sleep than when awake
c) Is usually worse when the person is tense or stressed
d) Usually stops when they activate another part of the body (e.g. foot-tapping or performing alternate movements of hands)
e) All of the above

165. Psychotropic drugs may modify hormone levels. Which of the following are true statements of demonstrated effects?

a) Narcotics can stimulated luteinizing hormone (LH) and testosterone secretion
b) Amphetamines reduce secretion of human growth hormone (HGH)
c) MAO inhibitors can block ovulation
d) Antipsychotic agents lower serum prolactin (PRL)
e) All of the above are true

Answers overleaf

163. b)

Resistance is an unwillingness, conscious or unconscious, to discuss material dealing with serious emotional conflicts, for fear of shame, rejection or anxiety. Secondary gain factors may also foster a resistance and preference to hold on the symptoms. *Projection* is an attribution of one's own feelings, wishes, or conflicts to others; *repression* is unconsciously keeping significant mental content out of consciousness, whereas *suppression* is doing this consciously. *Denial* is acting and thinking as if part of reality were not true.

CTP pp. 137-8. *CPM* pp. 20-21, 515-6. *GP* p. 564.

164. c)

a) No, the buccolinguomasticatory triad is described. There are usually sucking, smacking lip movements, cheek puffing, rolling, thrusting or 'fly-catching' movements of the tongue; and 'cud-chewing' and lateral jaw movements.

b) No, the movements disappear during sleep.

c) Yes, the movements are usually worse when under stress or tension.

d) No, they are often worse when another part of the body is active, and

e) is thus false.

CPM pp. 480-4. *GP* pp. 531-3.

165. c)

a) No, narcotics may lower LH and testosterone levels.

b) No, amphetamines stimulate HGH secretion.

c) Yes, MAO Inhibitors, and Reserpine, can block ovulation.

d) No, antipsychotics, dopamine-receptor blocking agents, raise serum PRL.

e) No.

166. Surveys of the mental health of the general population show that the percentage of people who can be classified as free of psychiatric symptoms is about:
   a) 5%
   b) 20%
   c) 45%
   d) 75%
   e) 95%

167. Which variety of schizophrenia is most likely to show an early onset, gradual deterioration, social isolation, and is not usually associated with hallucinations and delusions?
   a) Paranoid
   b) Catatonic
   c) Hebephrenic
   d) Simple
   e) Schizo-affective

168. Characteristic features of borderline personality disorder include:
   a) Transient, reversible psychotic episodes
   b) Systematic delusions
   c) Sublimation as the typical defence mechanism
   d) Consistently cooperative relationships with staff
   e) Superficial and transient interpersonal relations

Answers overleaf

166. b)

Only some 20% of the population is free of psychiatric symptoms. The often cited Midtown Manhattan study found only 18% symptom-free, 36% having mild symptoms, and 46% with moderate to incapacitating symptoms. The Stirling County, Canadian study found similar proportions affected.

CTP Chap. 5, pp. 97-102. *CPM* pp. 61-2.

167. d)

Simple schizophrenia, one of the varieties described by Eugen Bleuler, is characterized by early onset, gradual deterioration, social isolation, and absence of hallucinations and delusions.

CTP pp. 321-2. *CPM* p. 174. *GP* pp. 358-9.

168. a), e)

Relations vacillating between transient, superficial and intense, dependent, but full of manipulation and unreasonable demands, are typical; as are brief psychotic episodes under stress. Systematized delusions (b) are not typical, nor is sublimation (c) a typical defense—splitting and primitive types of projection are commoner; (d) is certainly incorrect, as stormy, ambivalent and highly disturbed relations with staff are typical.

Kernberg O. F. (1975); Mack J. E. (1975); Masterson J. F. (1976). *CTP* pp. 487-490. *CPM* pp. 387-9.

169. Which of these are typical of the hyperventilation syndrome?
a) Increased P_{CO_2}
b) Paraesthesia
c) Respiratory acidosis
d) Decreased cerebral blood flow
e) Increased free ionized calcium

170. Stupor may occur in:
a) Petit mal
b) Gjessing's periodic catatonia
c) Depression
d) Catatonic schizophrenia
e) All of the above

171. Recognized features of hypomania and mania include:
a) Absence of depression
b) Euphoria
c) Irritability
d) Decreased psychomotor activity
e) Hallucinations

Answers overleaf

169. b), e)

a) No, there is reduction of P_{CO_2}, and respiratory alkalosis.
b) Yes, paraesthesia, numbness and tingling, especially of lips and fingertips, are typical.
c) No, with reduction in P_{CO_2}, there is respiratory alkalosis.
d) No, there is decrease in free ionized calcium in relation to the alkalosis.
e) Yes, related to the alkalosis.

CTP, Chap. 24.6, pp. 620-1. *CPM* pp. 373-4. *GP* pp. 181-2.

170. e)

a) Yes, in the uncommon situation of petit mal status. The EEG shows continuous spike and wave forms.
b) Yes, with very slow waves in the EEG during reaction phases.
c) Yes, in the now uncommon severe retarded depression.
d) Yes, and therefore
e) is the correct response

CTP p. 314. *CPM* p. 171.

171. b), c), e)

a) No, periods of depression may occur during hypomanic or manic episodes, and there is a real suicide risk.
b) Yes, with expansiveness and often infectious humour.
c) Yes, and anger if and when thwarted.
d) No, increased psychomotor activity is typical.
e) Yes, especially in more severe, psychotic forms of mania, hallucinations do occur in as many as 25% of such cases, though they are usually brief and non-compelling.

CTP pp. 714-5. *CPM* pp. 143-9. *GP* pp. 331-4.

172. The IQs of a group of medical students are distributed according to the normal curve, with a mean of 115 and a standard deviation of 10. This means that:

a) 50% will have IQs less than 115
b) 5% will have IQs less than 105
c) 2.5% will have IQs greater than 135
d) 2.5% will have IQs greater than 125
e) 10% will have IQs less than 70

173. Drugs which may produce hostile or violent reactions, alone or in combination with others, include all of these EXCEPT:

a) Amphetamines
b) Diazepam
c) Barbiturates
d) Frusemide
e) Phencyclidine

174. In hypoparathyroidism, with low serum calcium, recognized psychiatric features may include all of these EXCEPT:

a) Irritability
b) Cyclic mood disturbance
c) Stupor
d) Paranoid psychosis
e) Lethargy

Answers overleaf

172. a), c)

With a normal, Gaussian distribution, the mean ±1 standard deviation covers 68% of the scores, mean ±2 SD covers 95%, and mean ±3 SD covers 99.73% of scores.

Swinscow T. D. (1980).

173. d)

a), b), c), e) All produce such reactions, and d) is the only exception. Hostility and violent reactions are seen significantly associated with ingestion of amphetamine, barbiturates, phencyclidine, diazepam, alcohol and marijuana.

Tinklenberg J. R., Stillman R. C. (1979).

174. c), e)

(a), (b), (d) These, as well as arousal, excitment, hyperactivity and irritability, are seen in experimental animals when CSF calcium is reduced by ventricular infusion of citrate, EDTA, or artificial CSF low in calcium.

(c) and (e) these features are more typical of hyperparathyroidism and increased calcium levels. In experimental animals, sedation and catatonic states are induced by increased ventricular calcium.

Carmen J. S., *et al.* (1980).

175. The classical epidemiological study showing an inverse relationship between social class and mental illness (that is, showing a higher prevalence in lower socioeconomic classes) was that of:
   a) Harry Stack Sullivan
   b) A.B. Hollingshead and F.C. Redlich
   c) Karl L. Kahlbaum
   d) Erich Fromm
   e) K. Abraham and K. Horney

176. In the episodic dyscontrol syndrome:
   a) The patients commonly experience an aura prior to the violent episode
   b) The patients usually show no remorse for their actions
   c) The treatment of choice is a benzodiazepine
   d) Abnormal neurological findings are very rare
   e) Treatment is rarely successful

177. Pathological excitement may occur in:
   a) Depression
   b) Mania
   c) Catatonia
   d) Delirium
   e) All of the above

Answers overleaf

175. b)

In 1958 August Hollingshead and Frederick Redlich published *Social Class and Mental Illness*, based on studies carried out in New Haven. These also showed that middle and upper class patients tended to use outpatient clinics and private practitioners, and lower class patients made more use of hospitals. Sullivan, Horney, and Fromm are neo-Freudians and Abraham an early psychoanalyst. Kahlbaum, in the 1860s, coined the term 'cyclothymia'.

CTP p. 11 Sullivan pp. 152-155, Abraham p. 9; Horney pp. 9, 150; Kahlbaum pp. 345, 375; Fromm, p. 11.
CPM pp. 63-64, Horney pp. 25-26; Fromm 26-27; Sullivan 24-25.

176. a)

a) Yes, there may also be other episodes of altered consciousness, such as staring spells, between attacks.
b) No, and this may be of diagnostic significance. They often express profound remorse, finding their attacks repugnant and foreign, ego-dystonic, and voluntarily seek help.
c) No, violence can be aggravated or precipitated by benzodiazepines.
d) No, 50% have at least one 'soft sign' (e.g. ataxia, astereognosis, memory impairment, etc.). Over 60% have EEG abnormalities, nonspecific or temporal spiking.
e) No, anticonvulsants like phenytoin may produce a substantial reduction in frequency and severity of attacks. Lithium has been suggested; and in severe cases, neurosurgery such as amygdalectomy has helped.

CTP pp. 587-9. *GP* p. 119.

177. e)

a) Yes, in agitated depression, the patient being obviously miserable.
b) Yes, the patient may be cheerful, or irritated and angry.
c) Yes, in catatonic excitement. The patient may show senseless and purposeless violence.
d) Yes, the delirious patient may show ill-directed overactivity.

CPM p. 171.

178. In obsessive–compulsive neurosis:

a) The patient usually responds with surrender and acceptance
b) The obsessions are regarded by the patient as ego-alien
c) Flooding may be a useful treatment technique
d) Drugs are of relatively little value in treatment
e) Thought-stopping may help to control obsessive ruminations

179. What effect does acute alcohol intoxication have on sleep in normal subjects?

a) Increases REM (rapid eye movement) sleep
b) Suppresses REM sleep
c) Reduces overall duration of sleep
d) Abolishes slow wave sleep
e) No systematic effects on sleep

180. Which case identification method produces the lowest proportion of patients with mental disorder in primary care settings?

a) Biochemical assay
b) Physician survey
c) Standardized psychiatric interview of patients
d) Patient symptom questionnaire
e) Medical record diagnosis audit

Answers overleaf

178. b), c), e)

a) No, the usual response is apprehension, annoyance and resistance.
b) Yes, they experience the obsessions as absurd, irrational, abnormal and ego-dystonic.
c) Yes, flooding in imagination and *in vivo* can be helpful.
d) No, clomipramine (Anafranil) for example, the tricyclic antidepressant, may be useful in the treatment of obsessional neurosis.
e) Yes, this may be a useful technique.

CTP Chap. 19.3, pp. 438-6. *CPM* pp. 395-6. *GP* pp. 309-10.

179. b)

Acute alcohol intoxication suppresses REM sleep, increases slow wave sleep at onset of sleep, but has no effect on growth hormone secretion patterns during sleep.

CTP pp. 527-528. *CPM* p. 53.

180. e)

Comparing case identification methods, it has been found that routine medical record audit identifies mental disorders in some 1-6% of patients; physician surveys around 10-22%; patient symptom questionnaires 20-36%; and patient standardized psychiatric interview techniques about 22-27%. Patients thus identified tend to use general medical services at significantly higher frequencies than other patients

181. Beta-endorphins attach themselves to which receptors in the brain

a) Benzodiazepine
b) Dopamine
c) Opiate
d) Histamine H_1
e) Muscarinic

182. Kurtosis refers to:

a) An effect of acute alcohol intoxication on red blood cells
b) A variety of tremor seen in Hartnup disease
c) An inborn error of metabolism
d) The shape of the peak of a frequency polygon
e) A type of chromasomal non-dysfunction

183. Anxious behaviour very similar to that which is produced by a frightening situation, has been provoked by electrical stimulation of the:

a) Hypothalamus
b) Nucleus/pocus/ceruleus
c) Cerebellum
d) Cerebral cortex
e) Vagus

184. Benign intracranial hypertension can be associated with:

a) Addison's disease
b) Hyperparathyroidism
c) Anaemia
d) Sagital sinus thrombosis
e) Oral contraceptives

Answers overleaf

181. c)

Beta-endorphins attach to opiate receptors.

Costa E., Trabucchi M. (1978); Usdin E. *et al.* (1979); Kline N. (1981).
CTP pp. 503, 598. *CMP* pp. 14–5, 48–9. *GP* pp. 517.

182. d)

Kurtosis, a statistical term, refers to the sharpness of the peaks in a frequency polygon. A sharp-peaked curve shows leptokurtosis, while a very flat curve is platokurtic.

Downie N. M., Starry A. R. (1977); Robson C. (1951).

183. b)

In experimental situations, electrical stimulation of the locus ceruleus has produced a response which mimics anxiety and fear.

Redmond D. E. *et al.* (1976).
CPM pp. 40. *GP* pp. 278–9.

184. a), d), e)

Benign intracranial hypertension can be associated with Addison's disease, hypoparathyroidism (not hyperparathyroidism), polycythaemia (not anaemia), sagittal sinus thrombosis, oral contraceptives and chlortetracycline administration. The mechanism underlying these effects is not understood.

185. Which of the following are NOT associated with Turner's syndrome?

a) Male gender identity
b) Female gender identity
c) XO chromasome pattern
d) Short stature
e) XXY chromasome pattern

186. The stimulant effect of alcohol on the nervous system is due to:

a) Stimulation of brain stem centres
b) Stimulation of cortical neurones
c) Depression of inhibitory brain stem centres
d) All of the above
e) None of the above

187. Which of the following findings would be convincing evidence that blood in a CSF sample was from a pre-existing subarachnoid haemorrhage, and not due to a traumatic lumbar puncture?

a) Large number of red blood cells in the CSF
b) Crenation of the red blood cells on microscopy
c) Macrophages laden with red cells
d) Xanthrochramia of the supernatant fluid after centrifugation
e) All of the above

188. In regard to child development, the concept of critical periods refers to:

a) Ages at which the child is especially sensitive to criticism
b) Emotional crisis that are necessary and functional for personality development
c) Periods during which children are highly critical of their parents
d) Developmental events that must occur at a particular time
e) None of the above

Answers overleaf

185. a), e)

Male gender identify and an XXY karyotype is typical of Klinefelter's syndrome.

CTP p. 32, 547, 861. *CPM* p. 404. *GP* p. 55.

186. c)

The stimulant effect on behaviour is due to depression of inhibitory centres in the brain stem.

187. c), d)

Several hours are needed for macrophages to become laden with red cells, and sufficient lysis of cells to produce xanthochromia similarly takes same hours. Thus either of these findings would suggest that the blood was from a haemorrhage preceding the lumbar puncture. The relative number of red cells, or crenation of the cells, are irrelevant in making this distinction. The relatively greater osmolarity of CSF in relation to the red cells can produce crenation of even those cells resulting from a traumatic puncture.

188. d)

This is the correct definition of the concept of critical periods. A variety of processes, including closure of the palate, social bonding, and maximal development of particular physical skills, all need to begin by a certain age or they will not occur, or will be faulty.

CTP pp. 834–7.

189. Which of these features are typical of anxiety?
a) Evidence of genetic predisposition
b) Evidence of parasympathetic nervous system arousal
c) The pupils are constricted
d) Increased plasma free fatty acids
e) Decreased basal skin conductance

190. Typical symptoms of normal-pressure hydrocephalus include:
a) Intermittent headaches
b) Dementia
c) Urinary and faecal incontinence
d) Ataxia
e) Blurred vision

191. The Stockholm syndrome is characterized by:
a) High blood pressure with low salt content of the sweat
b) The hostage develops strong positive feelings for the hostage taker
c) Hypomagnesaemia following diuretic usage
d) Mental retardation, contralateral hemiplegia and epilepsy
e) Paranoia on the part of the hostage-taker

Answers overleaf

189. a), d)

a) Yes, there is a general population prevalence of around 5%; and incidences of around 50% in children of patients, 15% in parents and sibs; there is 41% concordance in monozygotic, and 4% in dizygotic twins.
b) No, the signs are of sympathetic, adrenergic, arousal—sweating, tachycardia, and increased cardiac output, pulse and blood pressure.
c) No, the pupils are dilated, due to sympathetic arousal.
d) Yes, following increased insulin release.
e) No, there is increased basal skin conductance and sweating.

CTP Chap. 19.1, pp. 426–31. *CPM* pp. 396–7. *GP* pp. 276–92.

190. b), c), d)

The mental deterioration of dementia, ataxia and incontinence forms a typical triad of presentation of normal pressure hydrocephalus. Headaches are not characteristic, nor is blurred vision.

CTP p. 418. *CPM* pp. 317–8. *GP* pp. 195–6.

191. b)

The Stockholm syndrome (named after a famous example occurring during a 1974 Stockholm bank robbery) describes one of the psychological sequelae of becoming the hostage of a kidnapper, terrorist or criminal; in which the captive develops significant positive feelings toward the captor (which may be reciprocated) and negative feelings toward the authorities responsible for rescue.

Ochberg F. M. (1980).

192. Prolonged apnoeic reactions following ECT, given using modern techniques, is due to:

a) Galactosaemia
b) The effects of an abnormal blood-brain barrier
c) An abnormal response to the anaesthetic
d) Deficiency of pseudocholinesterase
e) Deficiency of phosphoribosyl transferase

193. A man in his 70s has been complaining of lethargy and anhedonia, and the presentation is reminiscent of depression. His daughter, who accompanies him, says that he seems to ignore the left side of his body in his daily activities at home and while dressing and combing his hair. He denies this firmly. One should suspect a diagnosis of:

a) Frontal lobe lesion
b) Right temporal lobe lesion
c) Right parietal lobe lesion
d) Left cerebellar lesion
e) Left pontine lesion

194. To which of the following constituents are drugs NOT likely to be bound?

a) Plasma albumen
b) Cellular proteins
c) Phospholipids
d) Nucleoproteins
e) Free ions

Answers overleaf

192. d)

Prolonged apnoea, occurring in around 1 in 3000 cases, is due to prolonged action of the muscle relaxant succinylcholine (Scoline) in the presence of a deficiency of pseudocholinesterase.
CTP Chap. 29.5, pp. 818–22. *CPM* p. 533.

193. c)

This symptom—denying or ignoring one side of the body—is called anosognosia. It is seen most often in people with lesions in the non-dominant parietal lobe. There may be other deficits in spatial recognition and integration of body image. Lesions in the dominant parietal lobe may produce the Gerstmann syndrome with finger agnosia, dyscalculia, agraphia and right-left disorientation.
CTP pp. 240, 247. *CPM* p. 351.

194. e)

Free ions as such are not involved in the binding of drugs, which may otherwise be bound to plasma albumen, cellular proteins, phospholipids or nucleoproteins.

195. Treatable causes of dementia include:
a) Alzheimer's disease
b) Normal-pressure hydrocephalus
c) Pellagra
d) Hypothyroidism
e) Arteriosclerotic dementia

196. A circadian rhythm has one cycle about every:
a) 8 hours
b) 24 hours
c) 90 minutes
d) 30 days
e) 365 days

197. Thigmotaxis in humans is:
a) A tendency to stay close to the wall in large unfamiliar open places
b) A preference for lying prone when stressed
c) A tendency to avoid brightly lit areas
d) An increase in serum viscosity in relation to climatic changes
e) None of the above

Answers overleaf

195. b), c), d)

Hypothyroidism can be treated with thyroxine, pellagra can be treated with niacin, and normal-pressure (communicating) hydrocephalus with ventriculo-atrial shunting. Alzheimer's disease and arteriosclerotic dementia are not reversible.

CTP pp. 392–8. CPM 273–83. GP pp. 69–127.

196. b)

A circadian rhythm has a cycle about every 24 hours. Human circadian rhythms can be altered by lithium and oestradiol. There are sleep/wake, activity, temperature and cortisol cycles, for example.

CPM pp. 128–30.

197. a)

A taxis is an unlearned orienting response relating to specific stimuli, and the human tendency to keep close to the wall or boundary in unfamiliar open places is an example, called thigmotaxis. The tendency to avoid brightly lit areas is also a taxis, but most noticeable in the albino rat.

198. The differential diagnosis of anorexia nervosa includes:
a) Shaman's syndrome
b) Sheehan's syndrome
c) Simmond's disease
d) Simon's disease
e) Occult neoplasm

199. Which of the following are not recognized side-effects of diphenylhydantoin (Epanutin/Dilantin)
a) Gum hypertrophy
b) Hirsutism
c) Ataxia
d) Cough
e) Peripheral neuropathy

200. Why is L-dopa used in the treatment of Parkinson's disease, rather than dopamine?
a) Dopamine is too rapidly metabolized to noradrenaline (norepinephrine)
b) Dopamine does not cross the blood-brain barrier
c) L-dopa has no side-effects
d) D-dopa, which would be ideal, is not stable in solution
e) It increases brain levels of dopa decarboxylase

Answers overleaf

198. b), c), e)

a) Shaman's syndrome: No (whatever it is). A shaman is a tribal healer, but has nothing to do with anorexia nervosa.

b) Sheehan's syndrome: Yes, though very rare, this variety of acute pituitary infarction following childbirth can produce a superficially similar clinical picture.

c) Simmond's disease: Yes, this rare variety of panhypopituitarism may resemble anorexia nervosa, but not closely.

d) Simon's disease: No, whatever it might be.

e) Occult neoplasm: Yes, though improbably, this may produce a superficially similar picture.

But patients with (b), (c) or (e) will not *behave* like anorexics in their attitudes to food, weight and body image, or in their capacity for deceit.

CTP Chap. 24.2, pp. 607–12. *CPM* pp. 250–2. *GP* pp. 163–8.

199. d)

Cough is not a recognized side-effect of diphenylhydantoin. These include gum hypertrophy, hirsutism, ataxia, peripheral neuropathy, diplopia, rash and lymphadenopathy.

CTP p. 416. *CPM* pp. 149, 203, 372, 466.

200. b)

Dopamine does not cross the blood-brain barrier. L-dopa can, and is then converted to dopamine within the central nervous system.

CTP pp. 407–8, 417. *CPM* pp. 133–4, 483. *GP* pp. 98–9.

201. Which of these are features typical of catatonic stupor?
 a) Physiological measures indicate low 'arousal'
 b) Amnesia for the period of stupor is unusual
 c) ECT may be helpful therapeutically
 d) Recovery from stupor is slow and uncommon
 e) The EEG shows a waking record

202. Which of the following statements about sexual abuse of children are true?
 a) Sexual abuse of children occurs rarely
 b) Sexual abuse occurs only with children of school age or older
 c) By definition, sexual abuse is the occurrence of intercourse between an adult and a child
 d) Sexual abuse usually occurs when a stranger takes advantage of an unprotected child
 e) Both boys and girls are victims of sexual abuse

203. Which area of the brain produces pleasure and elation on electrical stimulation?
 a) The amygdala
 b) The caudate nucleus
 c) The septal region
 d) The cingulate gyrus
 e) The reticular system

Answers overleaf

201. b), c), e)

Physiological measures indicate high arousal; amnesia for the period of stupor is unusual; ECT can be therapeutically effective; recovery from the attack is likely, and not usually very slow, though the underlying disease process continues; the EEG does show a waking record.

CTP pp. 243, 267. *CPM* pp. 170–1. *GP* p. 361.

202. e)

a) False, it is probably the most under-reported and under-diagnosed type of child abuse. Though there are no reliable figures of actual incidence, the rapid increase in reported cases has led to significantly higher estimated incidence.

b) False, victims of sexual abuse range from infants to those at the legal age of consent.

c) False, sexual abuse includes any variety of sexual activity with a child, including manual, oral or genital contact and sexual harrassment.

d) False, the abuser is usually known to the child, and may be a close relative, mother's boyfriend or close friend of the family, babysitter or someone else entrusted with the child's care.

e) True, both boys and girls are sexually molested both by older children and adolescents and by adults. It is true, however, that a majority of reported cases involve abuse of females by males. Sexual abuse may present as acting-out behaviour by the child, lying or stealing, truancy, promiscuity, running away from home; or physical complaints like headache, fatigue, dizziness, or abdominal pains.

CTP p. 724–5.

203. c)

The septal region often produces pleasurable sensations on electrical stimulation in humans, and both humans and animals will repeatedly administer such stimulation to themselves, given the opportunity. Septal stimulation can also produce erections and orgasms in humans and animals.

204. **Typical symptoms of withdrawal from heroin and other opiates include:**
   a) Sweating
   b) Constipation
   c) Lacrimation
   d) Bradycardia
   e) Cramps

205. **Primary process thinking is:**
   a) Prominent in the psychoses
   b) Primitive and non-rational
   c) Typical of a normal infant
   d) Prominent in dreams
   e) All of the above

206. **The commonest psychiatric disturbance associated with Cushing's syndrome is:**
   a) Anxiety neurosis
   b) Mania
   c) Organic brain syndrome
   d) Depression
   e) Psychosis

Answers overleaf

204. a), c), e)

Withdrawal symptoms include sweating, lacrimation and rhinorrhoea, cramps and muscle aches, fever, yawning, tachycardia and diarrhoea. These may begin within a few hours after the last dose, and reach a maximum within 24 to 48 hours. The experience is generally unpleasant but not very dangerous in itself.

CTP p. 506. *CPM* pp. 229–32. *GP* pp. 221–6.

205. e)

Primary process is contrasted with secondary process thinking which is more mature, rational and adult with a good relation to external realities and acceptance of delay of gratification.

206. d)

Mania and organic brain syndrome/delirium may occur, but depression is the most common problem and may be the most severe.

CTP pp. 627–8, 688. *CPM* pp. 245, 359–60. *GP* p. 131.

207. What is the average concordance rate for bipolar manic-depressive illness in monozygotic twins?
   a) 90%
   b) 75%
   c) 50%
   d) 25%
   e) 10%

208. Early symptoms of lithium carbonate toxicity include:
   a) Muscle twitching
   b) Haematuria
   c) Slurred speech
   d) Drowsiness
   e) Hypothyroidism

209. Compulsive water drinking (psychogenic polydipsia) may be distinguished from diabetes insipidus, because in compulsive water drinking:
   a) Plasma osmolality is higher than normal
   b) Urine concentration is greater after fluid deprivation than after vasopressin
   c) Urine flow increases after infusion of hypertonic saline
   d) Administration of vasopressin relieves thirst
   e) Onset of polydipsia is before polyuria

Answers overleaf

207. b)

Combining several studies, the average concordance rate for bipolar manic-depressive illnesses in monozygotic twins is, on average, 75%. In dizygotic twins and other siblings it is 20% to 25%, substantially higher than in the general population.

CTP pp. 26–8. *CPM* pp. 64, 122. *GP* p. 53.

208. a), c), d)

When blood levels of lithium exceed 2 mg per litre, CNS signs of toxicity begin to emerge—muscle twitching, slurred speech, drowsiness; and later coma, increased muscle tone, and convulsions. Haematuria does not occur and hypothyroidism, while it might occasionally be related to lithium use, is not a sign of toxicity.

CTP pp. 827, 406, 828. *CPM* pp. 457–66, 566–7. *GP* pp. 550–1.

209. b), e)

a) No, plasma osmolality is lower than normal in polydipsia (under 275 mosmol/kg water); high (over 290 mosmol/kg water) in diabetes insipidus. Normal is 280 ± 6.

b) Yes, the opposite is true of diabetes insipidus.

c) No, it *decreases* in polydipsia and in normal individuals; there is little change in diabetes insipidus.

d) No, it does not relieve thirst—it causes headache, bloating, nausea, vomiting and irritability, in polydipsia and normal people. Patients with diabetes insipidus feel better after administration of vasopressin.

e) Yes, polydipsia usually begins before polyuria in psychogenic polydipsia; polydipsia usually begins after polyuria in diabetes insipidus.

CPM pp. 458–59.

210. Selective deprivation of dream sleep produces:
a) No observable effect
b) Temporary psychotic states
c) Diffuse ego boundaries
d) Specific memory deficits
e) Subsequent compensatory increase in dreaming

211. The research of Masters and Johnson shows that the first physiological response to any variety of sexual stimulation in women is:
a) Clitoral erection
b) Tachycardia
c) Erection of the nipples
d) Vaginal lubrication
e) Carpopedal spasm

212. A major reaction to nalorphine, with sweating, running nose, yawning, tears, dilated pupils and restlessness, suggests:
a) An abstinence syndrome secondary to cocaine addiction
b) An abstinence syndrome secondary to heroin addiction
c) Dextropropoxyphene toxicity
d) Amphetamine toxicity
e) All of the above

Answers overleaf

210. e)

People deprived of dream sleep may be more irritable and distractable than those deprived of non-dream sleep, but the principle effect is a subsequent compensatory increase in the proportion of dream sleep during the sleep that follows such deprivation.

211. d)

The physiology is complex, but vaginal lubrication is usually the first sign of arousal. This is not due to secretions, but a transudate produced by vasocongestion resulting from marked dilation of the venous plexus surrounding the vagina.

Masters W. H., Johnson V. E. (1970).
CTP pp. 563–4.

212. a)

An abstinence syndrome like this would occur in heroin addicts, on receiving nalorphine.

CTP p. 500. *GP* pp. 220–1.

213. The Ganser syndrome occurs in:
a) Avitaminosis
b) Senility
c) Prisoners awaiting trial
d) Depression
e) Schizophrenia

214. Common features of anorexia nervosa include:
a) Increased BMR
b) Lanugo
c) Mirror-gazing
d) Increased libido
e) Hypotension

215. Which of these statements does NOT describe a consequence of occlusion of the anterior cerebral artery
a) Motor dysphasia on the dominant side
b) Cortical, flaccid, weakness of the opposite leg
c) Cortical sensory loss on the opposite leg
d) Grasp reflex
e) Ipsilateral weakness and spasticity of the upper body

Answers overleaf

213. c)

This clinical presentation, with a childish, ludicrous performance on clinical testing, with paralogia—'approximate answers' is typical. It is a variety of malingered craziness described in prisoners awaiting trial.

CTP pp. 654–5. *CPM* pp. 423–4. *GP* pp. 297–8.

214. b), c), e)

a) No, *decreased* BMR is more typical.
b) Yes, this variety of body hair is common in anorexia nervosa.
c) Yes, there is a distorted body image and preoccupation with one's image, often with mirror-gazing.
d) No, there is decreased interest in sex.
e) Yes, as signs of cachexia, there may be hypotension, bradycardia, constipation, dependent oedema and hypothermia.

CTP Chap. 24.2, pp. 607–12. *CPM* pp. 250–2. *GP* pp. 165–6.

215. e)

a) Yes, from involvement of the precentral gyrus of the frontal lobe.
b) Yes.
c) Yes, because of involvement of the superior surface of the cerebral cortex.
d) Yes, from frontal lobe involvement.
e) No, *contralateral* weakness and spasticity may occur if Heubner's artery (the medial striate artery) branch is occluded, affecting the anterior limb of the internal capsule, carrying fibres supplying the upper part of the body and extra pyramidal nuclei.

216. Which of the following statistical tests deal with rank correlations?

a) Student's T
b) Kendall's tau
c) Spearman's rho
d) Chi-square test
e) All of the above

217. Which of these drugs are NOT potentially dangerous in porphyria?

a) Tetracycline
b) Propoxyphene hydrochloride
c) Phenobarbital
d) Phenytoin
e) Sulphonamides

218. Which of these statements about the experience of depersonalization are NOT true?

a) The experience is delusional
b) The unreality feelings are pleasant
c) The unreality feelings are unpleasant
d) The unreality feelings relate to the self, the body and the world
e) The feelings clear on treatment with barbiturates

219. In childhood enuresis (bed-wetting) which of the following are true?

a) It generally occurs during REM sleep
b) It occurs in 50% to 60% of normal 4-year-olds
c) It is usually a sign of significant psychopathology
d) Treatment with imipramine may be useful
e) Behaviour therapy can aid bladder control

Answers overleaf

216. b), c)

Kendall's tau co-efficient, and the Spearman rank-order correlation co-efficient rho, deal with rank correlations. Student's t does not, expressing degree of confidence in the equality or difference between means. It is named after the pseudonym 'student' used by the man who devised it, when he described it in 1908. The Chi-square Test also does not deal with rank-orders.

Downie N. M., Starry A. R. (1979); Robson C. (1973).

217. a)

Tetracycline is not potentially dangerous in porphyria. Delta-ALA-synthetase is a necessary enzyme in the formation of porphyrin precursors. Its activity is increased (with resultant increase information of porphyrins) by a variety of substances including these (phenobarbital, propoxyphene, phenytoin and sulphonamides) and also other barbiturates, glutethimide, meprobamate, tolbutamide, chloroquine, oestrogens, progesterone, griseofulvin and alcohol.

Massey E. W. (1980).
CTP pp. 421, 688. *CPM* p. 306. *GP* pp. 140–1.

218. a), b), e)

The experience of depersonalization is not delusional (the patient recognizes it as odd and 'false'), it is rarely felt to be pleasant, and does not respond to barbiturates.

CTP pp. 420–2. *CPM* p. 533. *GP* pp. 312–3.

219. d), e)

Enuresis occurs in 10% to 15% (rather than 50% to 60%) of normal 4-year-olds; it is not usually associated with significant psychopathology or physical anomalies; it occurs generally during non-rapid eye movement (NREM) sleep. Both imipramine and behaviour therapy may be beneficial.

CTP pp. 985–7. *GP* pp. 479–80.

220. The symptom complex characteristically shown by children deprived of their mother (and of an effective substitute) during their earliest years of life is called
   a) autism
   b) anaclitic depression
   c) stranger anxiety
   d) encopresis
   e) separation anxiety

221. Which of these antipsychotic drugs is the most strongly anticholinergic?
   a) Haloperidol (Haldol)
   b) Trifluoperazine (Stelazine)
   c) Thioridazine (Melleril)
   d) Thiothixene (Navane)
   e) Phenelzine

222. Studies of thyroid function in depression have demonstrated that:
   a) T^3 has no effect on the effectiveness of tricyclic antidepressants
   b) Thyroid-stimulating-hormone (TSH) response to thyrotropin-releasing hormone is heightened in some depressed patients
   c) Only male patients have shown an enhancing effect when small doses of T^3 were administered concurrently with a tricyclic antidepressant
   d) Most depressed patients are euthyroid by usual standards
   e) None of the above

Answers overleaf

220. b)

Infants deprived of mother or mother surrogate in early life show anaclitic depression. After initial vigorous protest, and then severe despair, a phase of detachment and withdrawal from interaction follows.

CTP p. 258. *CPM* p. 121.

221. c)

Thioridazine is the most strongly anticholinergic. Phenelzine is not an antipsychotic.

CPM p. 281.

222. d)

(a) Untrue, small doses of triiodothyronine (T^3) have been shown to significantly potentiate the therapeutic effects of tricyclic antidepressants (and TSH has shown a similar effect). But, contrary to statement (c), this effect has only been shown in *women* patients, so the response appears to be sex-related. Contrary to statement (b), TSH response to TRH is impaired in some depressed patients; (d) is true.

CPM p. 139.

223. The differential diagnosis of anxiety state includes all of these EXCEPT:
a) Phaeochromocytoma
b) Carcinoid syndrome
c) Hypothyroidism
d) Caffeinism
e) Withdrawal from sedative drugs

224. Which of these statements about the use of placebos are TRUE?
a) Placebos have no physiological effects
b) The use of placebos is inherently unethical
c) Placebos cannot be used without deceiving the patient
d) Placebos are only effective on psychologically determined symptoms
e) Placebo responders cannot be predicted by personality and psychological studies

225. The consistency of scores one person obtains on a test taken on different occasions is referred to as:
a) The modal response
b) The Kuder-Richardson score
c) The split-half score
d) The validity
e) The reliability

Answers overleaf

223. c)

Hypothyroidism is not a likely differential diagnosis. Phaeochromocytoma may produce episodic or sustained symptoms, with increased blood pressure, severe headache, flushing, and increased urinary catecholamines. Carcinoid syndrome tends to produce anxiety with itchy, flushed and blotchy skin, and increased 5-HIAA in urine. Caffeinism has a characteristic history. Withdrawal from sedatives, especially barbiturates or alcohol, can produce anxiety with clouding of consciousness as part of the withdrawal syndrome.

GP p. 271, 276–92.

224. e)

a) No, placebo action may produce some clear physiological effects, such as anti-tussive and anti-emetic effects.

b) and c) No, placebo treatment does not rely on deception for its effects, and is not unethical when properly used; even if many doctors misuse it in ways that at times border on the unethical.

d) A symptom or condition does not have to be psychological in origin to benefit from placebo response; and placebo response does not suggest that the symptom was faked, 'psychological', psychosomatic, or 'not real'.

e) Yes, there have been many attempts to identify a placebo-reactor type or personality, but with no consistent findings. The individual who responds to a placebo is not predictable or identifiable except by that response.

GP pp. 558–9.

225. e)

This consistency is called the reliability of the test.

226. A patient asks you whether there could be any problem if he mixes alcohol with diazepam. Your advice would be:

a) There is no problem with the combination as they have complimentary effects
b) Any problems will be negligible at a dose of less than 50 mg a day
c) Alcohol will decrease the side-effects of diazepam
d) Do not mix diazepam and alcohol: the combination can lead to unexpected increases in the effects of either
e) The combination increases the risk of cirrhosis

227. In Jungian analytical psychology, a person's outer representation of his conscious intentions and relations to the expectations of society is called the:

a) Ego
b) Archetype
c) Persona
d) Libido
e) Cathexis

228. Predictors of poor response to lithium prophylaxis in manic-depressive illness include:

a) Prior history of relapse while on lithium
b) Prior history of slow change of cycle
c) Severity of depressive episodes
d) Hallucinations and thought disorder during manic episodes
e) Relatively poor response to antidepressants

Answers overleaf

226. d)

Simultaneous use of diazepam with other CNS depressants, such as alcohol, is contraindicated and may also increase respiratory depressant effects. In addition, alcoholics like other substance abusers may be more likely to develop dependency problems. Alcohol has no helpful effects on diazepam side-effects; problems may well arise at doses below 40 to 50 mg per day. The combination has no effect on increasing predisposition to cirrhosis

227. c)

This is called the persona, a term which Jung used in a way similar to the sociological concept of social role.

CTP p. 161. *CPM* pp. 22-3. *GP* p. 36.

228. a), d)

a) Yes, prior history of relapse while on lithium suggests a prior response is likely.
b) No, previous *rapid* change of cycle is of poorer prognostic significance.
c) No, not relevant in this context.
d) Yes, this is indicative of worse prognosis.
e) No, not relevant in this context.

CTP Chap. 29.7, pp. 825-9. *CPM* p. 455.

The next eight questions are in an alternate format. Within each question, there is a set of items lettered, A,B,C, etc., and a set numbered 1,2,3 etc. For each lettered item, select the single numbered item that is most closely associated with it.

229. Link the names (A–E) with the appropriate number (1–5) of the concept with which that individual is associated

A. Jung
B. Freud
C. Adler
D. Lorenz
E. Moreno

1. The Id
2. Organ inferiority
3. Psychodrama
4. Archetypes
5. Imprinting

230. Which of the following rates (1–6) express the frequency of schizophrenia

A. In the general population
B. In siblings where one sib has schizophrenia
C. In identical twins where one twin has schizophrenia

1. 20% to 30%
2. 30% to 50%
3. 2% to 3%
4. 10% to 15%
5. Less than 1%
6. 18%

Answers overleaf

229. A-4, B-1, C-2, D-5, E-3

CTP Jung: p. 8, Chap. 8.3, pp. 160–1; Freud: Chap. 6, pp. 119–47 Adler: Chap. 7.1, pp. 148–50; Lorenz: p. 71; Moreno: p. 10; Psychodrama: Chap. 78.4, pp. 761–2.

CPM Jung: pp. 12–3, 22-3, Freud: pp. 11–2, 19; Adler: pp. 12, 24

GP Freud: pp. 21–30; Jung: pp. 30–1; Adler: pp. 31–2; Lorenz: p. 2; Moreno (p. 585).

230. A-5, B-4, C-2

A-5. General population incidence is less than 1%.
B-4. Where one sib has schizophrenia, the incidence in siblings is 10% to 15%.
C-2. Where one twin has schizophrenia the incidence in the other monozygotic twin is 30% to 50%.

CTP Chap. 2.1, pp. 23–33, p. 300. *CPM* pp. 162–163.

231. Match the following clinical descriptions (A-E) with the appropriate psychopathological description of the phenomena (1-5)

A. A patient is asked the name of the previous Prime Minister. He replies, 'Wilson'. He is asked the name of the present PM, and replies, 'Wilson. Sorry—I mean Wilson'
B. A patient experiences his thoughts as being foreign to him and under outside control
C. A patient sees a truck drive past and immediately identifies it as part of a drug-dealing conspiracy, endangering him.
D. A patient is asked: 'What's the colour of grass' He answers, 'White.' Asked the colour of snow, he replies 'Green'.
E. A patient calls a watch a 'clock vessel' and calls a lamp a 'relitivitous'.

1. Thought alientation
2. Vorbeireden, talking past the point, giving approximate answers
3. Perseveration
4. Neologism
5. Delusional perception

232. Match the names (A-E) to the treatment techniques (1-5) with the development of which these men are associated

A. Moniz
B. Cerletti
C. Meduna
D. Freud
E. Wolpe

1. Insulin coma therapy
2. Free association
3. ECT
4. Leucotomy
5. Behaviour therapy

Answers overleaf

231. A-3, B-1, C-5, D-2, E-4

Hamilton M. (1974).

Thought alienation—*CTP* pp. 295, 317; *CPM* pp. 168-9.

Vorbeireden and the Ganser syndrome: *CTP* pp. 654-5, *CPM* pp. 423-4.

Perseveration: *CPM* p. 171.

Neologism: *CTP* p. 314; *CPM* pp. 168-170.

Delusional perception or primary delusions: *CTP* pp. 237, 238, 311. *CPM* pp. 169-70.

232. A-4, B-3, C-1, D-2, E-5

Moniz and leucotomy: *CTP* Chap. 29.6, pp. 822-5.
Cerletti and Bini and ECT: *CTP* Chap. 29.5, pp. 818-2.
Meduna and insulin coma therapy: *CTP* pp. 829-31.
Freud and free association: *CTP* Chap 6, esp. pp. 122, 146, 728.
Wolpe and behaviour therapy: *CTP* p. 62, Chap. 28.2 pp. 743-7.
Free assoc: *GP* pp. 563-4.
Leucotomy: *GP* pp. 601-5.
Insulin coma: *GP* pp. 605-7.
Behavior therapy: *GP* pp. 572-5.

233. Match the following genetic terms (A–E) with the appropriate definition (1–5)

A. Variable expressivity
B. Polygenic transmission
C. Autosomal dominant
D. Autosomal recessive
E. Sex-linked dominant

1. A trait which appears only when the individual is homozygous for the gene
2. Multiple genes are essential contributions to one trait
3. The same gene may affect two different individuals to different degrees
4. Transmission by a gene located on a sex chromosome
5. A trait which will ordinarily be expressed if the relevant gene is present on either member of a chromosome pair

234. Match the following terms (A–E) with the appropriate illustrative clinical example (1–5)

A. Extracampine hallucinations
B. Reflex hallucinations
C. Autoscopy
D. Delusional zoopathy
E. Functional hallucinations

1. A patient is convinced that he is infested with creatures, though they cannot be seen by others
2. The patient sees someone standing behind him when he is looking straight ahead
3. A patient hears voices amidst the ticking of a clock
4. The patient sees himself and knows that it is himself, like a doppelganger
5. The patient feels a pain in her head when she hears other patients sneeze, and experiences these events as causally connected

Answers overleaf

233. A-3, B-2, C-5, D-1, E-4
CTP Chap. 2.1, pp. 24–32.

234. A-2, B-5, C-4, D-1, E-3

A-2. This is a hallucination beyond the limits of the sensory field concerned. It has no specific diagnostic significance, and may be hypnogogic, organic or schizophrenic in origin.

B-5. Here a stimulus in one sensory field is felt to produce a hallucination in another—a morbid variety of synaesthesia.

C-4. A phantom mirror-image, commonest in delirium, may occur in schizophrenia.

D-1. Often organic in origin, may be schizophrenic in origin.

E-3. An external stimulus causes a hallucination experienced as well as the stimulus, e.g. voices in birdsong or a running tap—seen in chronic schizophrenia. But *not* an illusion.

Hamilton M. (1974).
CTP pp. 657–658.

235. Match each clinical problem (A-E) with its primary clinical feature (1-5)

A. Couvade syndrome
B. Oneirophrenia
C. Gilles de la Tourette syndrome
D. Latah
E. Koro

1. Panic and fear that genital shrinking will lead to death
2. Male showing symptoms of pregnancy
3. Culture-bound disorder with echolalia and echopraxia
4. Acute psychotic state with dream-like clouding of consciousness
5. Involuntary tics and obscene utterances

236. Match the following terms (A-E) which have been used in studies of schizophrenia with the appropriate definition (1-5)

A. Pseudomutuality
B. Schism
C. Skew
D. Invalidation
E. Praecox feeling

1. An overt conflict, with covert dependence in a marriage
2. Denial or ignoring the perceptions or feelings of family members
3. A method by which a family system maintains a rigid or abnormal equilibrium
4. Lack of overt conflict, with convert hostility and centring around a pathological parent within a marriage
5. An intuitive experience by the physician that it is not possible to establish empathic rapport with the patient

Answers overleaf

235. A-2, B-4, C-5, D-3, E-1

Couvade: *GP* p. 33.
Gilles de la Tourette: *CTP* pp. 898–99. *CPM* pp. 420–1.
Koro: *CTP* p. 659. *CPM* pp. 70, 426. *GP* p. 412.
Latah: *CTP* p. 659, *CPM* p. 425. *GP* p. 412.
Tourette: *GP* p. 476–7.
Oneirophrenia: *CTP* p. 324. *CPM* p. 350.

236. A-3, B-1, C-4, D-2, E-5

Schism, Skew: *CPM* p. 64.
Praecox feeling: *CTP* p. 328.

237. The difference between the INCIDENCE and PREVALENCE of a condition is that:
   a) Incidence rates are always higher than prevalence rates
   b) Incidence includes only new cases, while prevalence includes new and existing cases
   c) Incidence includes cases that are no longer current
   d) Prevalence includes only new cases, while incidence includes only old cases
   e) Incidence is an older term, relatively rarely used now, for what we now call prevalence

238. In the elderly patient, sensory loss should be considered as a particularly important potential causative factor in:
   a) Obsessive–compulsive neurosis
   b) Hypochondriasis
   c) Paranoid reactions
   d) Alcoholic disorders
   e) Manic episodes

239. Which of these psychiatric diagnoses have been unequivocally shown to be associated with predictable dangerousness to other people?
   a) Schizoid personality
   b) Sociopathic personality
   c) Manic-depressive psychosis
   d) All of the above
   e) None of the above

Answers overleaf

237. b)

Incidence expresses the number of new cases; while prevalence expresses the commonness of cases, both new and old, in the community—the proportion of a population that has the condition at any one time.

CTP p. 99. *CPM* pp. 60–1..

238. c)

Paranoid reactions are not uncommon as a response to sensory loss in the elderly.

CTP pp. 116–7, and Chap. 42. *CPM* pp. 272–3 *and* Chap. 32.

239. e)

None of the conditions listed, or any other psychiatric diagnosis, has been demonstrated to be predictably related to dangerousness to others.

CTP pp. 712–3. *CPM* pp. 561–3. *GP* pp. 622–3.

240. Which of these conditions is associated with a 'port wine stain' or facial cutaneous angioma?
   a) Von Recklinghausen's disease
   b) Tuberous sclerosis
   c) Schilder's disease
   d) Sturge-Weber syndrome
   e) Friedrich's Ataxia

241. With regard to tricyclic antidepressants:
   a) Their therapeutic effect is usually noticeable within a week
   b) They should be continued for some months after improvement of the patient's condition
   c) Especially in elderly patients, they may precipitate glaucoma
   d) Dizziness is a relatively common side-effect
   e) Overdoses are rarely fatal

242. Typical clinical features of hypomania include all of the following EXCEPT:
   a) Relatively acute onset
   b) Insomnia
   c) Sustained, affable cheerfulness
   d) Poorly sustained attention
   e) Lack of insight

Answers overleaf

240. d)

The 'port wine stain' is typical of the Sturge–Weber syndrome. It is probably due to an irregularly dominant gene, and includes a facial naevus within the area of distribution of the fifth cranial nerve, buphthalmos, and mental retardation.

CTP p. 862. *CPM* p. 409. *GP* p. 443.

241. b), c), d)

The therapeutic effect general requires ten days to two weeks; and overdose is quite frequently fatal.

CTP Chap. 29.2, pp. 789–7. *CPM* pp. 442–1. *GP* pp. 540–5.

242. c)

Sustained affability and cheerfulness is not typical of hypomania. The mood is labile, and the patient may show quick temper, anger, aggression and sadness.

CTP pp. 369–70. *CPM* pp. 143–9. *GP* p. 333.

243. The two tumour sites which are the commonest sources of metastases to the brain are:

a) Lung and colon
b) Colon and rectum
c) Rectum and ovary
d) Uterus and ovary
e) Breast and Lung

244. Which of the following is NOT a neurohormone, neuroregulator or transmitter synthesized by neurones?

a) Ceruloplasmin
b) Serotonin
c) Gamma-aminobutyric acid
d) Acetylcholine
e) Adrenaline (epinephrine)

245. The subtypes of dementia praecox described by Kraepelin include:

a) Catatonic
b) Paranoid
c) Hebephrenic
d) Chronic undifferentiated
e) Pseudoneurotic

Answers overleaf

243. e)

Breast and lung are the tumour sites which most commonly result in brain metastases.

Lishman W. A. (1978); Gilroy J., Meyer J. S. (1979). *CPM* pp. 352–3.

244. a)

Ceruloplasmin is not a neurohormone, regulator or transmitter. It is involved in the metabolism and carriage of copper in the blood. Very low levels occur in Wilson's disease (hepatolenticular degeneration).

CTP p. 858. *CPM* pp. 305–6.

245. a), b), c)

'Undifferentiated' is a later concept, as is 'pseudoneurotic', first described in 1949 by Hoch and Polatin.

Kraeplin's classification: *CTP* p. 298; *CPM* pp. 102–3.
Undifferentiated: *CTP* p. 322.
Pseudoneurotic: *CTP* pp. 323–4. *CPM* p. 175. *GP* p. 339.

246. A token economy system uses all of the following principles and techniques EXCEPT:
- a) Operant conditioning
- b) Positive reinforcement
- c) Shaping
- d) Prompting
- e) Flooding

247. Arrest of personality development at a stage short of uniform adult mature independence is called:
- a) Regression
- b) Suppression
- c) Fixation
- d) Retrogression
- e) Disassociation

248. Characteristic features of grief and bereavement include all the following EXCEPT:
- a) Feelings of guilt
- b) Expressed desire for psychiatric help
- c) Feelings of anger and hostility
- d) Somatic symptoms
- e) Preoccupation with memories of the deceased

Answers overleaf

246. e)

Flooding is the only principle or technique not used within a token economy system.

CTP Chap. 28.2, pp. 743–747. *CPM* p. 179.

247. c)

Such an arrest of personality development is called 'fixation'.

CTP pp. 123–8.

248. b)

Expressed desire for psychiatric help is uncommon and uncharacteristic, though fear of going mad may be disturbing.

Simpson M. A. (1979).
CTP pp. 693–4. *CPM* p. 543. *GP* pp. 322–3..

249. Regarding *folie à deux*:

a) Successful treatment usually requires separation of the participants in the folie
b) It is also known as pseudomutuality
c) It involves a psychosis shared between two people
d) It occurs when the separation–individuation phase of development is incomplete
e) Usually one of the participants is more actively disturbed while the other is a more passive follower

250. Pseudocyesis is usually associated with:

a) Abdominal enlargement
b) Menstrual disturbances
c) A common history of stillbirth
d) Other signs of malingering
e) None of the above

251. In a young woman patient, you find her pupils react poorly to light and slowly to accommodation, pupillary reactions to drugs are normal, and her knee jerks are absent. Would you:

a) Suspect a frontal tumour?
b) Suspect Adie's syndrome?
c) Expect to find positive history of syphilis?
d) Suspect Wernicke's encephalopathy?
e) Suspect cervical spondylosis?

Answers overleaf

249. a), c), e)

Folie à deux is a shared paranoid delusional system arising in a close relationship between a dominant paranoid individual and a more dependent and suggestible partner, living together in relative isolation.

CTP p. 349, 655-66. *CPM* p. 424. *GP* p. 363.

250. a), b)

Pseudocyesis is a 'false pregnancy'.

Enoch M. O., Trethowan W. H. (1979).

251. b)

The findings described would be typical of Adie's syndrome.

252. The 'revolving-door' syndrome

a) is otherwise known as the Schultz–Robinson syndrome
b) is a sign of cerebellar–vestibular dysfunction
c) refers to the cyclical re-admission of institutionalized patients
d) is an innovative exchange system between divisions in a chronic psychiatric hospital
e) is preferable to 'closed-door' or 'open-door' policies

253. Which of these psychological mechanisms are considered to be involved in the formation of phobic symptoms?

a) Displacement
b) Denial
c) Splitting
d) Regression
e) Avoidance

254. Unwanted side-effects of chlorpromazine include:

a) Hypertension
b) Photosensitivity
c) Weight loss
d) Lactation
e) Sleeplessness

Answers overleaf

252. c)

The term refers to the cycle by which institutionalized patients are discharged from chronic hospitals, and then re-admitted via hospital emergency rooms to chronic hospitals. It may generate impressive 'statistics' for 'patient care', though patients simply rotate between components of the system without adequate care.

CPM pp. 65–6.

253. a), e)

Displacement and avoidance are believed to be important mechanisms in the formation of phobic symptoms.

CTP Chap. 19.2, pp. 432–8. *CPM* pp. 392–5. *GP* p. 27.

254. b), d)

Photosensitivity, breast swelling and lactation are significant side-effects. Hypotension, weight loss, drowsiness and somnolence are other side-effects, as opposed to alternatives a), c) and e).

CTP Chap. 29.1, pp. 781–9. *CPM* pp. 469-72. *GP* pp. 521–6.

255. The incidence of a disease may be estimated from:
a) The number of cases in each age group, diagnosed in a hospital each year
b) The proportion of hospital beds occupied by patients with the disease
c) The proportion of people with the disease in a random sample of the population
d) The number of new cases occurring each year in a defined population
e) Mortality rates, if the case fatality ratio is high

256. Which of these statements about delusions are true?
a) They constitute reality for the patient
b) They usually resolve when factual proof of their falseness is presented
c) They are fixed false beliefs
d) They are commonly shared by others
e) All of the above

257. In Huntington's chorea:
a) It is transmitted by a single autosomal dominant gene
b) The gene has an almost 100% manifestation rate, so 100% of an affected person's children will develop the disease
c) The onset of symptoms is usually in early childhood
d) Choreiform movements are typical early signs
e) Gross personality change may occur

Answers overleaf

255. d), e)

Swinscow T. D. (1980).
CTP p. 99. *CPM* pp. 60–1.

256. a), c)

CTP pp. 237–8. *CPM* p. 90. *GP* p. 349.

257. a), d), e)

Only some 50% of the children of a patient with Huntington's chorea will ultimately develop the disease, and the onset of symptoms is usually between 25 and 55 years of age.

CTP pp. 29, 418. *CPM* pp. 50, 276, 335–7. *GP* pp. 96–7.

258. A week ago, a 68-year-old man with Parkinsonism was started on L-dopa and benzhexol. He has become confused and disoriented, and this morning tried to drink from a vase of flowers. This situation could be caused by:

a) L-dopa
b) Benzhexol
c) Neither drug
d) Either drug
e) His Parkinsonism

259. Delirium in association with glossitis, and with disturbance of vibration sense, is compatible with the diagnosis of:

a) Pernicious anaemia
b) Porphyria
c) Wernicke's encephalopathy
d) Myxoedema
e) Wilson's disease

260. Research studies may compare two or more cohorts. To be comparable, cohorts should share:

a) The same year of birth
b) Passage through the same time period
c) Common place of residence
d) Exposure to the same pathogens
e) Common medical history

Answers overleaf

258. d)

Either drug, L-dopa or benzhexol, could cause the clinical picture described.

CTP pp. 407, 417, 783. *CPM* pp. 133–4, 483.

259. a)

This clinical presentation is compatible with a diagnosis of pernicious anaemia.

CTP p. 688.

260. b)

Passage through the same period of time by both cohorts would be necessary.

Robson C. (1973); Walizer M. H., Wienir P. L. (1978); Downie N. M., Starry A. R. (1977).

261. Characteristic features of Gilles de la Tourette syndrome include:
- a) Sudden involuntary episodes of sleep
- b) Sudden involuntary movements
- c) Sudden involuntary utterances
- d) Sudden involuntary urination
- e) Coprolalia

262. A mixing of cells of differing genetic types in the same individual organism is called:
- a) Heterochromia
- b) Dimorphism
- c) Mosaicism
- d) Heteromorphism
- e) Heterogeneity

263. Classic psychoanalytic varieties of psychological defence mechanisms include all of the following EXCEPT:
- a) Repression
- b) Regression
- c) Sublimation
- d) Reaction formation
- e) Titration

Answers overleaf

261. b), c), e)

CTP pp. 256, 656–7, 896, 898–9. *CPM* pp. 420–1. *GP* pp. 476–7.

262. c)

263. e)

Titration is not one of the defence mechanisms.

CTP pp. 135–8. *CPM* pp. 20–1, 515–6. *GP* 26–9.

264. The extent to which a measurement process, such as a psychological test, truly assesses the trait it purports to assess is called:
   a) Objectivity
   b) Validity
   c) Reliability
   d) Efficiency
   e) Standard error

265. Hepatolenticular degeneration (Wilson's disease) is treated with:
   a) High copper diet
   b) Anticholinesterases
   c) Vitamin B_{12}
   d) Penicillamine
   e) Folic acid

266. The hypertensive crisis associated with MAOI treatment
   a) is usually fatal
   b) is more frequent with phenelzine than with tranylcypromine
   c) occurs with foods with high tyramine content
   d) should be treated with phentolamine
   e) should be treated with reserpine

Answers overleaf

264. b)

Swinscow T. D. (1980); Robson C. (1973); Walizer M. H., Wienir P. L. (1978); Downie N. M., Starry A. R. (1977).

265. d)

Penicillamine is the appropriate treatment for Wilson's disease.

CTP pp. 424, 688, 857. *CPM* pp. 305–6, 413. *GP* p. 448.

266. c), d)

(a) False, the reaction is rarely fatal, though it is very unpleasant, and it is not more common with phenelzine (b). As to (e), it should never ever be treated with reserpine. As reserpine depends on MAO for its hypotensive action, its use can make the situation worse.

CTP pp. 721–3. *CPM* pp. 439–40. *GP* pp. 539–40.

267. A major advantage of group therapy over individual psychotherapy is that it is:
   a) Less hard work for the therapist
   b) Allows the patient to try new ways of relating to others in a protected social environment
   c) A safe technique in the hands of untrained therapists
   d) Deeper interpretations of the patient's behaviour can be given and accepted far more easily
   e) Free of transference and counter-transference problems

268. With regard to patients attending a general practice and having recognizable psychiatric disturbance:
   a) The commonest varieties of problem are anxiety and depression
   b) Acute schizophrenia is seen relatively commonly
   c) They will make up around 20% to 30% of the patients attending the GP
   d) Most need to be referred to a psychiatrist
   e) Most will be referred to a psychiatrist

269. Antipsychotic drugs in low doses
   a) Are generally safer than benzodiazepines
   b) Have no significant autonomic side-effects
   c) Can be effective in treating anxiety
   d) Do not cause tardive dyskinesia in anxious patients
   e) Have a low potential for substance abuse

Answers overleaf

267. b)

Bion W. H. (1959); Lieberman *et al.* M. A. (1973) Rogers C. (1971).
CTP Chap. 28.4, pp. 750–761. *CPM* pp. 206–207. *GP* pp. 575–9.

268. a), c)

(b) Acute schizophrenia is uncommon; (d) most patients can be treated very adequately by the GP and do not need to be referred to a psychiatrist and (e) are not so referred.

CTP Chap. 26.4, pp. 702–3.

269. c), e)

As antipsychotic drugs may indeed cause tardative dyskinesia in anxious and other patients, (d) is not correct.

CTP Chap. 29.1, pp. 771–89. *CPM* pp. 469–88.

270. In phenylketonuria (PKU):
  a) It is due to a single autosomal dominant gene
  b) It is due to deficiency of the enzyme phenylalanine hydroxylase
  c) The child shows hypotonicity and hyporeflexia
  d) The child typically has brown eyes and dark hair
  e) The Guthrie test is of diagnostic value

271. The 'four As' of schizophrenia described by Eugen Bleuler:
  a) Are not found to occur significantly in any other disorder
  b) Include ambivalence and disorder of affect
  c) Include autism and loosening of associations
  d) Include avoidance and akathisia
  e) Are basically the same as Schneider's 'first rank' symptoms

272. Recently identified pepides which may be morphine-like neurotransmitters in the brain are:
  a) Vasopressins
  b) Prolactins
  c) Substance P
  d) Somatostatins
  e) Enkephalins

Answers overleaf

270. b), e)

The enzyme phenylalanine hydroxylase, absent or deficient in PKU, is essential for oxidising phenylalanine into tyrosine. Its lack leads to accumulation of phenylalanine. It is due to a recessive gene. The child shows hypertonicity and hyper-reflexia, and typically has blue eyes and fair hair.

CTP p. 853. *CPM* p. 405. *GP* pp. 444–6.

271. b), c)

These constitute Bleuler's 'four A's'.

CTP pp. 309–10. *CPM* p. 35.

272. e)

Correct, as the question refers to enkephalins or endorphins.

CTP pp. 503, 598. *CPM* pp. 14–5, 48–9, 165, 178, 248.

273. An electroenephalographic (EEG) pattern of a slow round wave followed by a quick sharp spike at 3 cycles per second is usually found in:
   a) Psychomotor epilepsy
   b) Grand mal epilepsy
   c) Petit mal epilepsy
   d) Meningioma
   e) Subdural haematoma

274. Generally, the EEG in delirium shows:
   a) Diffuse slowing
   b) Diffuse fast activity
   c) High voltage, fast activity
   d) Localized occipital slowing
   e) Generalized low amplitude spikes

275. The patient on lithium therapy may be especially prone to toxic effects under all of the following circumstances EXCEPT:
   a) If elderly
   b) If taking a low sodium diet
   c) If taking a thiazide diuretic
   d) If suffering from diarrhoea
   e) If suffering from hypothyroidism

Answers overleaf

273. c)

The 3-per-second wave and spike pattern on the EEG is typical of petit mal epilepsy.

CTP pp. 413–4. *CPM* p. 368. *GP* pp. 102, 112.

274. a)

Diffuse slowing in the EEG is typical in delirium.

CTP Chap. 18, pp. 388–391. *CPM* pp. 268, 272.

275. e)

Toxic effects of lithium are no more likely in someone suffering from hypothyroidism. A benign goitre may develop during long-term administration of lithium, and hypothyroidism may eventually occur—but toxic effects are not more likely. The other conditions listed can make a patient more prone to toxic effects which are more likely if the person (a) is elderly; (b) is on a low sodium diet (as lithium concentrations in the body are balanced by sodium and an adequate salt intake is needed); (c) if taking a thiazide diuretic, for similar reasons; and (d) if suffering from diarrhoea (if loss of salt and water is significant).

CTP Chap. 29.7, pp. 825–9. *CPM* pp. 451–69. *GP* pp. 550–1.

276. Behaviour therapy for the treatment of agoraphobia may include all of the following techniques EXCEPT:
   a) Systematic desensitization
   b) Flooding
   c) Aversive therapy
   d) Attention to reinforcement contingencies
   e) Family therapy

277. Features of amphetamine abuse generally include all of the following EXCEPT:
   a) Constricted pupils
   b) Anorexia
   c) Delusions of persecution
   d) Insomnia
   e) Visual hallucinations

278. With the use of benzodiazepines in the treatment of epilepsy, significant problems may include:
   a) Ataxia
   b) Tolerance to the anticonvulsant effects
   c) Excess sedation at the requisite doses
   d) Any of the above
   e) None of the above

Answers overleaf

276. c), e)

Wolpe J. (1973).
CTP Chap. 28.2, pp. 743–7, *and* pp. 236, 434–5. *CPM* pp. 393–4. *GP* pp. 289–9.

277. a)

Pupils are usually dilated, not constricted. The others are frequent features of amphetamine abuse.

CTP pp. 405, 515–6. *CPM* pp. 216–8. *GP* pp. 229–30.

278. d)

Appropriate answer, as any of these problems may complicate the use of benzodiazepines in treating epilepsy.

CTP p. 416. *CPM* pp. 489–492.

279. Gregory Bateson is associated with the 'double bind' hypothesis to explain aspects of:

a) Hysteria
b) Autism
c) Obsessive-compulsive neurosis
d) Involutional melancholia
e) Schizophrenia

280. Causes of mononeuritis multiplex include:

a) Trauma
b) Osteomalacia
c) Diabetes mellitus
d) Carcinoma
e) Polyarteritis nodosa

281. Clinically important physical dependence occurs with the following drugs:

a) LSD
b) Morphine
c) Cocaine
d) Amphetamine
e) Cannabis

Answers overleaf

279. e)

CTP p. 11, Chap 13.4, pp. 302-9. *CPM* p. 64, 159-60, 167-8. *GP* p. 352.

280. c), d), e)

Other causes include leprosy, sarcoidosis and rheumatoid disease.

Walton J. N. (1977).

281. b)

The other drugs do not cause physical dependence.

CTP Chap. 21, pp. 496-43. *CPM* Chap. 10, pp. 213-35. *GP* pp. 219-41.

282. Eight weeks after giving birth, a young woman complains of loss of libido, fatigue, tearfulness and poor appetite. Appropriate interventions would include:

   a) No treatment except brief reassurance
   b) Prompt treatment with a tricyclic or phenothiazine
   c) Involvement of the husband in helping his wife
   d) Practical help in managing the baby
   e) Investigation of hormone levels

283. The interpretation of a shadow on the wall as being another person in the room, is an example of:

   a) Paranoia
   b) Delusion
   c) Hallucination
   d) Illusion
   e) Idea of reference

284. Chloral hydrate, used to induce sleep:

   a) Resembles the barbiturates in its effects
   b) Resembles alcohol in its effects
   c) Has little effect on REM and stage IV sleep
   d) Acts by its effect on stage I of sleep
   e) Acts by conversion into L-tryptophan

Answers overleaf

282. c), d)

These would be appropriate interventions in such a case of postpartum 'blues'.

CTP pp. 380–2. *CPM* p. 247.

283. d)

CTP p. 251. *CPM* p. 90. *GP* p. 689.

284. c)

CTP pp. 405, 806. *CPM* p. 649.

285. Which of the following conditions are due to a dominant gene?

a) Schizophrenia
b) Phenylketonuria
c) Alzheimer's disease
d) Homocystinuria
e) Huntington's chorea

286. In various studies on stress, which of the following events is rated by most individuals as most stressful?

a) Loss of job
b) Death of a family member
c) Divorce
d) Serious medical illness
e) Marriage

287. A 'double blind' study of a treatment modality is one in which:

a) The experimental group receives the treatment and the control group receives a placebo
b) Neither observers nor subjects know the nature of the placebo
c) Neither observer nor subjects know which subject receives the treatment and which receives the placebo
d) Neither the experimental nor the control group knows the identity of the observers
e) The control group does not know the identity of the experimental group

Answers overleaf

285. e)

CTP pp. 29, 418. *CPM* pp. 50, 276, 335–7. *GP* pp. 96–7.

286. b)

CTP pp. 593, 693–4. *CPM* pp. 68–71. *GP* pp. 151–4.

287. c)

Robson C. (1973); Walizer M. H., Wienir P. L. (1978); Downie N. M., Starry A. R. (1977).
CPM p. 59.

288. Mr J. does not quarrel openly with his wife, but frequently angers her by forgetting promises and appointments with her, and neglecting his duties at home. Such behaviour would best be described as:

a) Reaction formation
b) Antisocial personality traits
c) Anal personality traits
d) Passive-aggressive personality traits
e) Introversion

289. Typical features of Korsakov's syndrome include all of the following EXCEPT:

a) Emotional lability
b) Brisk relexes
c) Chronic alcoholism
d) Disorientation in time and place
e) Confabulation

290. Which of these are often associated with anorexia nervosa?

a) Primary amenorrhoea
b) Lassitude
c) Abnormal gastric motility
d) Normal body image
e) Bulimia

Answers overleaf

288. d)

This vignette describes passive–aggressive personality traits, using passive, submissive behaviours as ways of expressing hostile or destructive feelings; exhibiting negativism, obstructions, inefficiency, sins of omission and similar responses.

CTP pp. 143, 493–4. *CPM* p. 384.

289. b)

Brisk reflexes are not typical in Korsakov's syndrome, where sluggish reflexes are more usual.

CTP pp. 395. *CPM* pp. 37, 197. *GP* pp. 209–10.

290. e)

Bulimia is often associated with anorexia nervosa; some describe 'bulimarexia' as a sub-type of this condition.

CTP pp. 265, 605. *CPM* p. 50. *GP* pp. 163–8.

291. The psychoanalytic concept of 'dream work' is:
   a) The process of transforming manifest dream content into latent content
   b) The process of transforming latent dream content into manifest content
   c) Energy expended in dreaming as estimated by EEG amplitude
   d) The number of underlying drives expressed in the dream
   e) None of above

292. Which of these statements about Down's syndrome are NOT true?
   a) The patient is prone to respiratory disease
   b) The patient typically shows a trisomy in group G (21-22)
   c) The patient is more likely to have congenital heart lesion than a normal child
   d) The patient is more likely to have been born to an older mother
   e) The patient has prominent epicanthic folds

293. Features of barbiturate withdrawal usually include all of the following EXCEPT:
   a) Insomnia
   b) Irritability
   c) Urinary frequency
   d) Tremor
   e) Anxiety

Answers overleaf

291. b)

Dream work was seen as using a range of mechanisms including symbolism, displacement, condensation, projection and secondary revision.

CTP pp. 131–32. *CPM* pp. 19, 22. *GP* p. 566.

292. b)

Robinson G. B., Robinson N. M. (1975), Stanbury J. *et al.* (1972). *CTP* pp. 31, 859–60. *CPM* pp. 403–4. *GP* pp. 449–52.

293. c)

CTP pp. 517–9. *CPM* 53, 215–6. *GP* pp. 237–40.

294. Causes of sudden blindness include:
a) Disc prolapse
b) Crigler–Najjar syndrome
c) Hysterical conversion
d) Methanol
e) Retrobulbar neuritis

295. The catastrophic reaction is seen in:
a) Populations responding to natural disasters
b) The use of hallucinogenic drugs in unfamiliar settings
c) Phobic patients confronted with the object or situation they fear
d) Brain-damaged patients in situations where they become aware of their deficits
e) Ailurophobia

296. Drugs which have NOT been shown to be effective in the management of some anxious patients include:
a) Propranolol
b) Beta-endorphin
c) Phenelzine
d) Meprobamate
e) Barbiturates

Answers overleaf

294. c), d), e)

Also acute glaucoma and vitreous haemorrhage.

Walton J. N. (1977).

295. d)

This is the best description of the catastrophic reaction. A demented patient, confronted with a task he cannot perform, may show anxiety, anger or rage.

296. b)

Beta-endorphin has not been shown to be effective in treating anxiety.

CTP pp. 503, 598; 426. *CPM* pp. 14–15, 48–9.

297. Stereognosis is the:

a) Knowledge of 'left' and 'right'
b) Ability to identify the direction from which a sound emanates
c) Ability to recognize shapes written on the skin
d) Appreciation of the form of an object by touch
e) Visual depth perception

298. Maxwell Jones made a significant contribution to the development of the concept of:

a) The amine hypothesis
b) Biofeedback
c) The therapeutic community
d) REM sleep
e) Gestalt therapy

299. Which of these statements about the elderly are true?

a) At age 65, average remaining life span exceeds 25 years
b) As an age group, the population 65 and over has the greatest prevalence of mental disorders
c) As an age group, the population 65 and older has the highest rate of suicide
d) The fastest growing age group in several Western countries is the population 75 and over
e) All of the above

300. Which of the following conditions is transmitted as a dominant trait?

a) Tay-Sachs disease
b) Gaucher's disease
c) Porphyria
d) Phenylketonuria
e) Galactosaemia

Answers overleaf

297. d)

Walton J. N. (1977).
CPM p. 350.

298. c)

Maxwell Jones is associated with the development of the therapeutic community concept.

Jones M. (1953).
CTP p. 11. *CPM* pp. 179–80. *GP* pp. 35, 382–4.

299. e)

Busse E., Blazer D. (1980); Birren J., Sloan R. R. (1980).
CTP Chap. 42, pp. 1017–22. *CPM* Chap. 32, pp. 639–53.

300. c)

CTP pp. 31, 421, 688. *CPM* pp. 403–10, p. 306.

REFERENCES

Ameer B., Greenblatt D. J. (1977). Acetaminophen. *Annals of Internal Medicine;* **87**:202-9.

American Board of Psychiatry and Neurology (1977). *Information for Examiners*: October 17-18 1977. Illinois, Evanston.

Anderson P. O. (1979). Drugs and breast feeding. *Seminars in Perinatology;* **3**,3:271-8.

Ayd F. J. (1973). Excretion of psychotropic drugs in human breast milk. *International Drug Therapy Newsletter;* **8**:33-40.

Bielsk R. J., Friedel R. O. (1976). Prediction of tricyclic antidepressant response: a critical review. *Archives of General Psychiatry;* **33**:1479-1489.

Bion W. H. (1959). *Experiences in Groups*. New York, Basic Books.

Birren J., Sloan R. R. (eds.) (1980). *Handbook on Mental Health and Aging*. New York, Prentice-Hall.

Blackwell B. (1979). Treatment adherence: a contemporary overview. *Psychosomatics;* **20**:27-35.

Bochner F., et al. (1978). *Handbook of Clinical Pharmacology*. Boston, Little, Brown.

Brain W. R. (1955) *Diseases of the Nervous System*. London: Oxford University Press.

Busse E., Blazer D. (ed.) (1980). *Handbook on Psychiatry and Aging*. New York, Van Nostrand.

Calesnick B. (1980). Tricyclic antidepressant toxicity. *American Family Physician;* **6**:104-107.

Cantwell D. (1975). *The Hyperactive Child: Diagnosis, Management and Current Research*. New York, Spectrum.

Carmen J. S., Crews E., et al. (1980). Calcium and Calcium-regulating hormones in the biphasic periodic psychoses. *Journal of Operational Psychiatry;* **11,1**:5-17.

Carrol B. J., Mendels J. (1976). Neuroendocrine regulation in affective disorder. In *Hormones, Behaviour and Psychopathology*. (Sachar E. J., ed.) New York, Raven Press.

Chess S., Hassibi M. (1978). *Principles and Practice of Child Psychiatry*. New York Plenum Press.

Costa E., Trabucchi M. (1978). *Review of the Endorphins*. New York, Raven Press.

CPM = Slaby A. E., Tancredi L. R., Lieb, J. (1971). *Clinical Psychiatric Medicine.* Philadelphia, Harper & Row

Crome P. (1980). Tricyclic antidepressant poisoning. *Hospital Update;* **6,**4:369–374

CTP = Kaplan H. I., Sadock B. J. (1981). *Modern Synopsis of the Comprehensive Textbook of Psychiatry III.* 3rd edn. Baltimore/London, Williams & Wilkins.

Downie N. M., Starry A. R. (1977). *Descriptive and Inferential Statistics.* New York/London, Harper & Row.

Editorial (1975). Paracetamol hepatotoxicity. *Lancet;* **2:**1189–1191

Enoch M. D., Trethowan W. H. (1979). *Uncommon Psychiatric Syndromes.* 2nd ed. Bristol, John Wright.

Erkkola R., Kanto J. (1972). Diazepam and breast-feeding. *Lancet;* **1:** 1235–1236.

Figley C. R. (ed.) (1978). *Stress Disorders Among Vietnam Veterans: Theory, Research and Treatment.* New York, Brunner/Mazel.

Flavell J. H. (1963) *The Developmental Psychology of Jean Piaget.* Princetown, N.J., Van Nostrand Co.

Freud A. (1946). *The Ego and the Mechanisms of Defense.* New York, International Universities Press.

Gilman A., Goodman L. S., Gilman A. (eds.) (1980). *The Pharmacological Basis of Therapeutics.* 6th ed. New York, Macmillan.

Gilroy J., Meyer J. S. (1979). *Medical Neurology.* 3rd ed. New York, Macmillan.

GP = Sim M. (1981). *Guide to Psychiatry.* 4th edn. London, Churchill–Livingstone.

Grinker R. R., Werble D., Drye R. C. (1968). *The Borderline Syndrome: A Behavioral Study of Ego Functions.* New York, Basic Books.

Hackett T. P., Cassem N. H. (1978). *Handbook of General Hospital Psychiatry.* St Louis, C. V. Mosby.

Hamilton M. (ed.) (1974). *Fish's Clinical Psychopathology.* Bristol, J. Wright.

Harden R. M., Brown R. A., Biran L. A., Dallas Ross W. P., Wakeford R. E. (1976). Multiple choice questions: to guess or not to guess. *Medical Education;* **10:**27.

Hatton, C. L., Valente S. M., Rink A. (1977). *Suicide: Assessment and Intervention* New York, Appleton–Century–Crofts.

Haynes, R. B., Taylor D. W., Sackett D. L. (1979). *Compliance with Therapeutic and Preventive Regimens.* Baltimore, Johns Hopkins University Press.

Jefferson J. W., Griest J. H. (1972). *Primer of Lithium Therapy.* Baltimore, Williams and Wilkins.

Jones M. (1953). *The Therapeutic Community: A New Treatment Method in Psychiatry*. New York, Basic Books.
Jung C. G. (1966). *Two Essays on Analytical Psychology*. Princeton, Princeton University Press.
Kaplan H. S. (1974). *The New Sex Therapy*. New York, Brunner/Mazel.
Kernberg O. F. (1975). *Borderline Conditions and Pathological Narcissism*. New York, Jason Aronson.
Kline N. (1981). The endorphins revisited. *Psychiatric Annals;* **11,4**: 27–35.
Kohut H. (1971). *The Analysis of Self: A Systematic Approach to the Psychoanalytic Treatment of Narcissistic Personality Disorders*. New York, International Universities.
Kupfer D. J., Spiker D. G., Coble P. A., et al. (1980). Depression, EEG, sleep and clinical response. *Comprehensive Psychiatry;* **21**:212–220.
Lieberman M. A., Yalom I. D., Miles M. B. (1973). *Encounter Groups: First Facts*. New York, Basic Books.
Lishman W. A. (1978). *Organic Psychiatry*. Oxford/New York, Oxford University Press.
Luborsky L., Singer B., Luborsky L. (1976). Comparative studies of psychotherapies: is it true that 'everybody has won and all must have prizes?' In *Evaluation of Psychological Therapies*. (Spitzer R. L., Klein D. F. ed.) pp 3–22. Baltimore, Johns Hopkins University Press.
Mack J. E. (ed.) (1975). *Borderline States in Psychiatry*. New York, Grune & Stratton.
Maletzky B. M. (1973). The episodic dyscontrol syndrome. *Diseases of the Nervous System;* **34**:178–185
Massey E. W. (1980). Neuropsychiatric manifestations of porphyria. *Journal of Clinical Psychiatry;* **41,6**:208–213.
Masters W. H., Johnson V. E. (1970). *Human Sexual Inadequacy*. Boston, Little, Brown.
Masterson J. F. (1976). *Psychotherapy of the Borderline Adult*. New York, Brunner/Mazel.
Melman K. L., Morelli H. F. (1978). *Clinical Pharmacology*. 2nd ed. New York, Macmillan.
Noyes R. (1979). Near-death experiences: their interpretation and significance. In *Between Life and Death*. (Kastenbaum R. ed.) pp. 75–88. New York, Springer.
Ochberg F. M. (1980). Victims of terrorism. *Journal of Clinical Psychiatry;* **41**:73–74.
Patrick M. T., Tilstone W. J., Reavey P. (1972). Diazepam and breast-feeding. *Lancet* **1**:542–543.

Paul S. M. (1981). The benzodiazepine receptor complex. *Syllabus and Scientific Proceedings*. American Psychiatric Association, 134th Annual Meeting, New Orleans, 1981, pp. 12-13.

Piaget J. (1929). *The Child's Conception of the World*. New York: Harcourt, Brace Jovanovich.

Piaget J. (1952). *The Origins of Intelligence in Children*. New York: International Universities Press.

Pinder R. M., Brogden R. N., Speight T. M., Avery G. S. (1977). Doxepin up-to-date: a review of its pharmacological properties and therapeutic efficacy. *Drugs;* **13**:161-218.

Post F. (1965). *The Clinical Psychiatry of Late Life*. Oxford: Pergaman Press.

Rapaport R. N. (1967). *Community as Doctor*. London, Tavistock Publications.

Redmond D. E. et al. (1976). Behavioural effects of stimulation of the *locus coeruleus* in the stump tail monkey. *Brain Research;* **110**:502.

Robinson G. B., Robinson N. M. (1975). *The Mentally Retarded Child*. 2nd ed. New York, McGraw-Hill.

Robson C. (1973). *Experiment, Design and Statistics in Psychology*. London, Penguin.

Rogers C. (1951). *Client-Centered Therapy*. Boston, Houston Mifflin.

Rogers C. (1970). *Carl Rogers on Encounter Groups*. New York, Harper.

Rosenbaum J. F. (1980). Psychotropic drugs and the cardiac patient. *Drug Therapy*; March: 79-88.

Scheinberg P. (1981). *Modern Practical Neurology*. 2nd ed. New York, Raven Press.

Schlesser M. A., Winokur G., Sherman B. M. (1980). Hypothalamic-pituitary-adrenal axis activity in depressive illness. *Archives of General Psychiatry;* **37**:737-743.

Secunda S. (1980). Doxepin: recent pharmacologic and clinical studies. *Proceedings of the American Psychiatric Association Annual Meeting*, San Francisco, 1980. 3 D.

Showalter C. V., Thornton W. E. (1977). Clinical pharmacology of phencyclidine toxicity. *American Journal of Psychiatry;* **134,11**:1234-1238.

Silverman J. J. et al. (1979). Clinical significance of tricyclic antidepressant plasma levels. *Psychosomatics;* **20,11**:736-746.

Simpson M. A. (1979). *The Facts of Death*. London/New York, Prentice-Hall.

Singer E. (1970). *Key Concepts in Psychotherapy*. New York, Basic Books.

Snyder S. H. (1979). Receptors, neurotransmitters and drug response. *New England Journal of Medicine;* **300**:465-472.

Stanbury J. B., Wyngaarden J. B., Fredrickson D. S. (ed.) (1972). *The Metabolic Bases of Inherited Disease.* 2nd ed. New York/London, McGraw-Hill.

Stevenson I., Greyson B. (1979). Near-death experiences: relevance to the question of survival after death. *Journal of the American Medical Association;* **242**:265-267.

Strain J. J., Grossman S. (1975). *Psychological Care of the Mentally Ill: A Primer in Liaison Psychiatry.* New York, Appleton-Century-Crofts.

Strauss J. S., Carpenter W. T. (1977). Prediction of outcome in schizophrenia. *Archives of General Psychiatry;* **34**:159-163.

Swinscow T. D. (1980). *Statistics at Square One.* 6th ed. London, British Medical Association.

Tinklenberg J. R., Stillman R. C. (1979). Drug use and violence. In *Violence and the Struggle for Existence.* (Daniels D., Gilula M., Ochberg F., eds.) pp. 327-365. Boston, Little, Brown.

Usdin E., Bunney W. E., Kline N. S. (1979). *Endorphins in Mental Health Research.* London: Oxford University Press; New York: Macmillan.

Vogel A. V., Goodwin J. S., Goodwin J. M. (1980). The therapeutics of placebo. *American Family Practitioner;* **July**:105-109.

Walizer M. H., Wienir P. L. (1978). *Research Methods and Analysis: Searching for Relationships.* New York/London, Harper & Row.

Walton J. N. (ed.) (1977). *Brain's Diseases of the Nervous System.* 8th ed. London/New York, Oxford University Press.

Wells C. E., Duncan G. W. (1980). *Neurology for Psychiatrists.* Philadelphia, F. A. Davis.

Wender P. H. (1971). *Minimal Brain Dysfunction in Children.* New York, Wiley.

Wolf, S. (1959). The pharmacology of placebos. *Pharmacological Review;* **11**:689-704.

Wolpe J. (1973). *The Practice of Behavior Therapy.* 2nd ed. New York, Pergamon Press.

Zukin S. R., Zukin R. S. (1979). Specific phencyclidine binding in rat central nervous system. *Proceedings of the National Academy of Sciences;* **76**:5372-5376.

FURTHER READING

Anderson J. (1976). *The Multiple Choice Question in Medicine*. Tunbridge Wells, Pitman Medical.
Bewley T., Mahapatra S. (ed.) (1980). *Handbook for Inceptors and Trainees in Psychiatry*. Royal College of Psychiatrists.
Fleming P. R., Sanderson P. H., Stokes J. F., Walton H. J. (1976). *Examinations in Medicine*. London, Churchill-Livingstone.
Hassall C., Trethowan W. H. (1978). Multiple choice examinations: their predictive value in the preliminary test and the membership exam. *Bulletin of the Royal College of Psychiatrists;* **June**:101–103.
Hubbard J. F., Clemans W. V. (1961). *Multiple Choice Examinations in Medicine*. Philadelphia, Lea & Febiger. (Reprinted 1968.)
Maleson F. G., Fink P. J., Field H. L. (1980). Board certification anxiety. *American Journal of Psychiatry;* **137**,7:837–840.
Sarnacki R. E. (1981). *Test-taking Skills: A Programmed Text for Medicine and the Health Sciences*. Baltimore, University Park Press.

SUBJECT INDEX

Opposite each subject appears the numbers of questions testing knowledge in that area.

Affective disorders: 4, 19, 27, 32, 34, 41, 55, 70, 82, 93, 99, 131, 154, 158, 170, 171, 177, 192, 206, 208, 222, 228, 241, 242, 266, 275
Aging: 11, 25, 63, 77, 143, 156, 164, 238, 258, 299
Alcoholism: 50, 66, 148, 179, 186, 226, 289
Analytic concepts: *see* Psychotherapy
Anxiety: 15, 20, 29, 49, 56, 61, 104, 124, 169, 176, 183, 189, 223, 226, 296

Biochemistry and Physiology: 1, 4, 15, 19, 23, 49, 67, 70, 114, 126, 134, 140, 148, 154, 155, 164, 165, 181, 183, 186, 194, 196, 197, 210, 221, 244, 270, 272

Child and Adolescent psychiatry: 12, 18, 36, 38, 45, 57, 59, 79, 89, 90, 94, 100, 111, 115, 138, 188, 198, 219, 220, 261, 270, 292
Consultation–Liaison psychiatry: 6, 7, 9, 12, 42, 62, 78, 86, 98, 105, 117, 124, 141, 153, 160, 174, 198, 206, 209, 217, 222, 238, 250, 258, 282

Depression: 4, 19, 34, 41, 55, 61, 70, 82, 93, 99, 117, 131, 154, 158, 170, 177, 192, 206, 207, 208, 222, 228, 241, 260, 275
Diagnosis: *see* Psychopathology
Drug dependence 12, 17, 22, 40, 48, 54, 107, 116, 204, 212, 277, 281, 293
Drug therapy: 4, 6, 15, 20, 25, 27, 29, 32, 34, 38, 41, 43, 46, 49, 56, 65, 66, 70, 74, 82, 85, 86, 95, 99, 104, 105, 114, 117, 119, 121, 124, 131, 133, 143, 145, 158, 164, 173, 194, 199, 208, 217, 221, 224, 226, 228, 241, 254, 266, 269, 275, 278, 284, 293, 296

Emergency psychiatry: 5, 43, 95, 116, 121
Epidemiology: 14, 71, 75, 84, 93, 166, 175, 180, 230, 237, 255, 268

Forensic psychiatry: 57, 68, 75, 120, 173, 191, 202, 231, 239

General psychopathology: *see* Psychopathology
Genetics: 59, 84, 93, 102, 185, 207, 233, 257, 262, 285, 300
Geriatric psychiatry: *see* Aging
Group therapy: *see* Psychotherapy

History of psychiatry: 30, 81, 132, 229, 232, 245, 271
Human sexuality: *see* Sexuality

Mania: 27, 32, 171, 177, 208, 228, 242, 275
Mental retardation: 18, 59, 71, 96, 102, 118, 185, 240, 270, 292

Neuroanatomy and Neurology: 3, 33, 37, 44, 58, 61, 72, 87, 89, 101, 113, 128, 134, 135, 139, 148, 149, 153, 162, 164, 170, 183, 184, 186, 187, 190, 193, 199, 200, 203, 215, 217, 218, 240, 243, 251, 259, 265, 272, 273, 274, 280, 294, 295, 297

Old age: *see* Aging
Organic mental disorders: 11, 25, 52, 77, 89, 128, 139, 150, 152, 174, 177, 193, 195, 200, 206, 209, 222, 234, 238, 243, 257, 259, 265, 273, 274, 278, 289, 295

Personality disorders: 16, 159, 168, 176
Physical treatments: 136, 150, 162, 192
Physiology and Biochemistry: *see* Biochemistry and Physiology
Psychoanalysis: *see* Psychotherapy
Psychological tests: 2, 63, 69, 80, 92, 125, 129, 264, 295
Psychology: 9, 24, 45, 53, 73, 79, 80, 83, 90, 92, 97, 111, 112, 122, 123, 125, 130, 132, 136, 138, 151, 155, 157, 161, 163, 172, 197, 203, 205, 224, 227, 229, 246, 247, 248, 253, 263, 279, 283, 286, 288, 291
Psychopathology: 8, 10, 12, 16, 28, 35, 48, 51, 55, 83, 97, 98, 109, 119, 126, 127, 142, 144, 167, 170, 175, 177, 178, 183, 205, 209, 210, 213, 214, 218, 220, 231, 234, 235, 236, 247, 248, 249, 250, 252, 256, 257, 261, 268, 279, 282, 283, 284, 285, 286, 290, 300
Psychosomatics: *see* Consultation-Liaison psychiatry
Psychotherapy: 13, 14, 21, 24, 26, 31, 47, 53, 76, 108, 110, 122, 123, 130, 132, 136, 147, 151, 157, 161, 163, 227, 229, 232, 246, 247, 252, 263, 267, 276, 291, 298

Schizophrenia: 8, 30, 39, 46, 60, 74, 81, 84, 94, 105, 106, 127, 133, 142, 152, 161, 167, 170, 177, 201, 205, 221, 230, 231, 234, 236, 245, 249, 254, 269, 271, 279
Sexuality: 42, 50, 62, 64, 75, 91, 140, 146, 153, 154, 202, 203, 211
Statistics: 103, 172, 180, 182, 216, 225, 255, 260, 287
Substance abuse: *see* Drug dependence
Suicide: 5, 43, 88, 99